CRITICAL PSYCHIATRY

CRITICAL PSYCHIATRY

The Politics of Mental Health

Edited by
DAVID INGLEBY

Pantheon Books, New York

LIBRARY OF CONGRESS CATALOGING IN PUBLICATION DATA

Main entry under title:

Critical psychiatry.

  Includes bibliographical references.
  1. Mental health policy—United States. 2. Mental
health policy—Europe. 3. Psychiatry—Philosophy—
United States. 4. Psychiatry—Philosophy—Europe.
I. Ingelby, David.
RC437.5.C75   362.2'042'0973   79-1886
ISBN 0-394-42622-3
ISBN 0-394-73560-9 (pbk.)

Grateful acknowledgment is made to the following for
permission to reprint from previously published material:

This selection, Introduction and "Understanding 'Mental
Illness' ": Copyright © 1980 by David Ingleby
"The American Mental Health Industry": Copyright © 1980 by
Joel Kovel
"Breaking the Circuit of Control": Copyright © 1980 by Franco
Basaglia. This translation Copyright © 1980 by Maria Grazia
Gianichedda, David Ingleby, Pia Bryant and Anna Maria
Brandinelli.
"French Anti-psychiatry": Copyright © 1977 by Sherry Turkle.
This chapter is based on material developed in *Psychoanalytic
Politics: Freud's French Revolution* by Sherry Turkle. © 1978
by Basic Books, Inc., Publishers, New York. Used with
permission.
"On the Medicalization of Deviance and Social Control":
Copyright © 1979 and 1980 by Peter Conrad
"Report from Norway": Copyright © 1980 by Svein Haugsgjerd.
"Towards a Critical History of the Psychiatric Profession":
Copyright © 1980 by Andy Treacher and Geoff Baruch

Contents

Introduction

The background of this book

Mental illness, we are told, is a major problem of our time. Most citizens of the West, even if they do not see it as *their* problem, are constantly reminded of its existence: charity appeals drum home the statistics – in Great Britain, one in nine men and one in six women can expect to enter a mental hospital, while 25 per cent of all hospital beds are occupied by mental patients. In the U.S.A., we read, doctors write 200,000,000 prescriptions for psychoactive drugs in the course of a single year.

But what exactly *is* this problem, and why do we seem so bad at solving it? According to most psychiatrists, it is a clinical problem like any other, which medical technology, in its relentless forward march, will eventually get rid of for us – provided the funds keep coming in. If we do not seem to have made much progress to date, that is because psychiatry is still an 'infant science'.

To many thinking people, though, there seems to be something wrong with this answer. Mental illnesses, by and large, do not *feel* like other illnesses – the 'symptoms' are not annoying externalities, like the spots on the face of the chicken-pox victim; on the contrary, they seem to be features of the very life a person leads, and they reach down to the core of the personality. And there is surely something irrational about such exclusive concentration on treatment of the symptoms, when in fact these supposed illnesses seem to be generated as an inevitable by-product of our way of life – so inevitable, that developing countries about to take up the Western way of life are advised to set aside ample provision in advance for its psychiatric casualties.[1]

Indeed, the technological solution has its critics even within psychiatry itself. Disagreements which have existed for over a century continue to smoulder, as the proponents of rival theories and treatments vie for supremacy: significantly, the best recent account of British psychiatry bears the title *Psychiatry in Dissent*.[2] Moreover, in the last two decades new voices have been heard challenging the leadership of the profession itself; the 'medical mandate' has been questioned, not only by the so called 'anti-psychiatrists', but by psychologists, social workers and social scientists who question whether the problems really have much to do with medicine in the first place. In this book we will try to take stock of the controversies both within the psychiatric profession and outside it.

All these controversies, however, have a peculiarly interminable quality: questions about what mental illness is, who should treat it, and how, have become such perennial ones as to raise the suspicion that they are not, in the last analysis, open to factual solutions at all. One premise shared by all the contributors to this book is that mental illness is, in fact, a *political* issue: we believe that instead of treating it simply as a problem of finding effective means to an agreed end, we must consider instead the fundamental disagreements about *ends* which underlie current controversies. These disagreements, we shall argue, concern the very concept of 'mental health' itself; is it sufficient, for example, to define health merely in terms of availability for work, or readiness to fulfil whatever role society has laid down for one? Is our society such, indeed, that 'normality' could ever be equated with sanity?

The idea that psychiatry is a political issue is, of course, one which was first brought into public view by the 'anti-psychiatrists' who gained prominence during the late 1960s – Laing, Cooper, Basaglia, Szasz and others. Each of these figures stood for a different approach, and all have therefore disowned the umbrella label of 'anti-psychiatry'; Laing's work led him into a therapeutic concern with fundamental existential issues, while for Cooper 'anti-psychiatry' was replaced by 'non-psychiatry', as the questions resolved themselves into more purely political ones. Basaglia sent his staff out of the hospital into the community at large; while Szasz denounced all these varieties of 'creeping socialism', and insisted that psychiatrists should return to a contractual relationship with the patient, aimed simply at promoting individual liberty. Yet despite their differences, all these figures were united in seeing the scientific image of psychiatry as a smokescreen; the real questions were: whose side is the psychiatrist on? what kind of society does he serve, and do we want it?

All the contributors to this book share that view, and all of us have been deeply influenced by the writings and activities that came to be called (however misleadingly) 'anti-psychiatry'. Nevertheless, the present volume is more than just a re-statement of the views of the 1960s:

the changed context in which we are writing today compels a fresh look at the problems.

We should recall that at the time when anti-psychiatry came into being, a well-nigh apocalyptic atmosphere had been created by the challenges to established authority coming from students, factory workers, civil rights activists, anti-Vietnam War protesters, and so on. To many, revolution seemed around the corner; neither political organization nor theoretical sophistication seemed necessary to bring it about, since capitalist society seemed to be falling apart of its own accord.

Capitalist society, however, pulled itself together again remarkably swiftly: and while the movements of the 1960s left some permanent changes in the landscape, revolutionary euphoria faded rapidly as the sheer monolithic strength of the established order became apparent. A chorus of 'We told you so' came from the traditional Left, which denounced 'the politics of subjectivity',[3] the substitution of rhetoric for theory, and the belief that changes in life-style could somehow usher in the new order without any change in basic economic power-structures. Anti-psychiatry in particular was left high and dry; although organizations it had created (such as the Philadelphia Association, the Socialist Patients' Collective, the Mental Patients' Union, etc.) carried on functioning, most of the Left no longer regarded psychiatry as an important issue – while orthodox psychiatry went on its way undented. Peter Sedgwick[4] spoke for many socialists when he argued that mental illness *was*, after all, a medical problem, and that anti-psychiatry's preoccupation with 'inner space' represented a flight from 'objective' political realities. The message about the political nature of psychiatry seemed to have fallen on deaf ears. Likewise among the psychiatric establishment, which responded with a spate of crude diatribes more or less on the level of 'PSYCHIATRY RULES OK'; subsequent developments in psychiatry – such as the establishment of a Royal College in Britain, and the integration of psychiatric units into general hospitals – have further strengthened the traditional alliance between psychiatry and physical medicine. As Joel Kovel writes in Chapter 2, 'brain research' is everywhere heralded as the key to progress, for all the world as though it had only just been invented.

In retrospect, then, the anti-psychiatry of the 1960s appears to be very much a phenomenon of the age: its vague theories, its detachment from traditional politics, and its disregard for strategy all seem to have condemned it – like flower-power – to wilt when the good vibes faded away. A much more hard-headed approach, both intellectually and politically, is required if the message of that movement is not to be completely lost today.

While the political climate of recession and retrenchment in the 1970s has discouraged practical initiatives in this area, certain intellectual developments promise to make a renewed attack on the problems a little easier. For one thing, it is possible to discern on the Left today a disillusionment with purely 'objective' approaches: in a sense, 'inner space' is very much on the agenda again, as many have realized that the contradictions of the capitalist system are both reflected in, and sustained by, the individual psyche. A good example of this is provided by the Women's Movement, where many recent writers have argued that the vicissitudes of being a woman are more than simply economic or legal ones; besides the 'objective' issues of pay and legislation, psychological questions have to be faced about the way women's roles are constructed and lived out.

In seeking to understand these often unconscious phenomena, feminists have turned inevitably to psychoanalysis:[5] and a radical reinterpretation of Freudian theory, stemming from such writers as Lacan in France and Habermas in Germany, has not only made this return to psychoanalysis possible, but has gained considerable stimulus from it in return. This cross-fertilization between Freudian and Marxist views is one feature of the present intellectual scene which was virtually absent – except in France – during the heyday of anti-psychiatry: as Sherry Turkle describes in Chapter 5, outside France 'anti-psychiatric stances implied anti-psychoanalytic ones'. Laing, for example, though his early work on the intelligibility of psychoses had clear origins in his psychoanalytic training, seemed to turn his back on this tradition entirely. Today, however, it seems less and less plausible to regard psychoanalysis purely as an instrument of conformity; while we can readily understand Laing's reasons for rejecting it, it is nowadays hard to see how any significant understanding of the social meaning of 'mental illness' could be achieved while turning a blind eye to psychoanalysis. The chapters by Ingleby, Kovel, Turkle and Haugsgjerd hopefully illustrate the truth of this.

Other recent intellectual developments are also relevant to our task. Fundamental to the anti-psychiatrists' claim that psychiatry was a political matter was their attack on its traditional sources of legitimation, medicine and science; before the politics of psychiatry could be uncovered, the spurious authority and impartiality it borrowed from medicine and science had to be dispelled. The medical profession had no business dealing with mental problems, it was argued, because the problems were not usually physical in essence; doctors were no better equipped than the rest of us – and sometimes a lot worse – to understand human predicaments. Science had only confused the issue because its fundamental premise, that people were like things and could be studied in the same way as things, was degrading and far-fetched.

At the time, unfortunately, few people who were not already convinced of their truth seem to have been converted by these arguments. Partly, no doubt, this was because they threatened too many vested interests; but one cannot help suspecting that it was also because the arguments themselves were not very thoroughly worked out. Ideas cannot be constructed in a vacuum, and there were at the time very few frameworks within which these particular ideas could be discussed. Over the last two decades, however, much sharper intellectual tools have been developed with which to criticize the traditional justifications of psychiatric theory and practice.

In the first place, studies in the history and sociology of medicine have brought forward many new ideas about the role of psychiatry: although the work of Foucault was available in the 1960s, the chapters by Treacher and Baruch, Kovel, and Conrad show how more recent research sheds new light on the domination of psychiatry by medicine, and on the part played by psychiatry as a social institution.

Secondly, the assumptions which psychiatry incorporates about what it is to study people 'scientifically' have come under heavy attack from many quarters. In sociology, for example, the notion that social facts are 'things' has raised objections ever since Durkheim propounded it at the turn of the century; in recent years it has lost all intellectual respectability. Both Anglo-Saxon and continental philosophy are – unusually – united in confirming the inappropriateness of natural-scientific methods and concepts to the study of people. Even in psychology, there has arisen since the 1960s a climate of disillusionment with 'scientific' methods amounting (it is often said) to a crisis. Thus, criticisms of psychiatric theory can be given far more intellectual weight today than was possible only a short while ago.

Lastly, a change has occurred in our understanding of science itself. The breakdown of traditional empiricist philosophies of science, combined with increasing public mistrust about scientists' aims, has complicated the notion of 'objectivity' and opened up a new discourse about the social and political roots of science. New accounts have been put forward (for example, by Habermas) of the relation between knowledge and interest, and the tacit biases of much research have been systematically uncovered. All this work has contributed to the present volume; witness, for example, the use that Chapter 1 makes of Kamin's work on intelligence-testing.

To summarize, the intellectual climate of today makes it much more feasible to aim at a cogent critique of psychiatry than it was when the anti-psychiatrists' arguments were formulated. In this book, we have made no more than a start on this critique, but hopefully the book itself will encourage a debate out of which better solutions can emerge. At times the reader may feel that we are excessively occupied with theoretical questions, but past experience shows that the task of theory-construction cannot be skimped, and this makes for hard reading. (Readers who dislike this emphasis, however, may prefer to leave the first chapter till the end.)

Finally, it is important to remember that psychiatry itself has undergone certain transformations which by themselves make new arguments necessary. Much of the moral impetus of anti-psychiatry came from its attack on the mental hospital as a place of segregation and confinement; but in recent years – largely for administrative rather than humane reasons – the traditional asylum has tended to be replaced by services providing 'community care', and by the deceptive concept of 'integration' (which means, of course, integration with the rest of the sick, not with the sane). While each Western nation has arrived at this policy in different forms and for different reasons, it is striking (and surely not mere coincidence) that they all arrived at it around the same time. (Compare, for example, the 1959 Mental Health Act in Britain, America's 1960 'Community Mental Health Centers' legislation, and the 1960 memorandum on 'sectorization' in France.) This changed situation calls for a new critique – not one which discovers a new theme in psychiatry, but one which shows how the same theme is present in both old and new incarnations.

The plan of the book

Having outlined the basic concerns of this book, it remains to describe how it is organized. The first chapter is rather more concerned with theory than the rest. It serves a double purpose: to classify the many different theories which have been put forward to account for mental illness according to the 'paradigms' underlying them, and to show how paradigms are selected for their practical and political usefulness rather than simply on the grounds of 'truth'.

In the first section, I argue first that the criticisms of orthodox psychiatry voiced in recent years are not criticisms of medicine as such, but of *positivism* – the paradigm of studying human beings as if they were things. The thorough critique of positivism recently developed by social theorists and philosophers bolsters up the anti-psychiatrists' view: that psychiatry's claim to impartial, objective authority is nothing but a smokescreen concealing a highly partisan position. 'Treating people as things' is not only a questionable methodological precept, but a highly objectionable policy. This policy, I argue, has to be understood as reflecting not the private attitudes of individual psychiatrists, but the social role which psychiatry has acquired in the course of its history.

In the second section, I examine the alternatives to positivist psychiatry which have been put forward, classifying these as 'interpretative' approaches. The simplest of these, the 'normalizing' approach, involves the view that so-called mental illnesses are actually meaningful responses to difficult situations, which a sympathetic application of common sense can easily make intelligible. (This, in fact, is the view usually associated with anti-psychiatry.) Though this view has revealed many ways in which mental 'symptoms' express the conflicts which people experience within their allotted social roles, I argue that in many conditions a 'residue' remains which is refractory to common-sense understanding: instead of reverting to the positivist view, that this residue is the meaningless outcome of *causal* processes, I examine the way it can be accommodated within the other major interpretative approach – psychoanalysis. Despite the methodological and political ambiguities of psychoanalysis, I conclude that Freud's concept of *compulsive action* is the third term necessary for understanding both the intelligibility of psychiatric symptoms, and the madness of normal life. (It also provides the word 'illness' with a new meaning, so that although we have rejected the traditional medical model, we may still distinguish between everyday and psychiatric problems.)

Thus, what the first chapter argues for is a kind of psychoanalytic environmentalism, in which mental illness is indeed seen as a response to the contradictions of our present society, but one which is only fully intelligible in terms of *unconscious* meanings. This corresponds to the view held by the other contributors to the book – though there are obvious differences between Conrad, Treacher and Baruch, and Basaglia on the one hand, and Kovel, Turkle and Haugsgjerd on the other, over the relative importance of the psychoanalytic component.

In both sections, I try to answer the obvious question of why there is so little scientific evidence available which might support or refute such a view of mental illness; the answer I propose is twofold. Firstly, theories of this sort do not fit in with psychiatry's mandate to change not society but the individual; they are not investigated because psychiatry quite literally has no *use* for them. Secondly, such evidence as we do have for this view does not satisfy the conventional criteria of 'scientific' research, because those criteria are not the appropriate ones to use when interpreting the social intelligibility of human action; we are not dealing with simply a different theory, but a whole different *paradigm*.

The remainder of the book surveys the state of psychiatry, and of movements critical of it, in different parts of the Western world. The intention here is not to provide an exhaustive account – notable omissions are West Germany and Latin America – but to bring out the essential similarities in the situation of all these countries, which have in common the capitalist mode of production. Psychiatry in Communist countries is beyond our scope, though one point should perhaps be made here to anticipate the inevitable objection that 'since the phenomena we are describing can also be found in Communist countries, they have nothing to do with capitalism as such'. To this we would argue that if such is indeed the case (and analogies are by no means easy to establish), it reflects more the embryonic state of socialism in the countries concerned than the innocuousness of capitalism.

We begin our survey, fittingly, in the United States of America. Joel Kovel, in 'The American Mental Health Industry', describes mental illness and psychiatry as two sides of the same coin – 'the psychologization of human difficulties'. Kovel considers the period 1905–10 to mark the critical period of transition towards 'psychologization': this period saw both the beginnings of 'late capitalism' (defined by the ascendancy of technology), and the high-water mark of American socialism – whose failure, Kovel asserts, dialectically explains the success of American psychiatry.

Having stimulated human potentialities, the problem for late capitalism was to channel them away from the drive for social transformation, and back into material production and consumption: the 'mental hygiene' movement proved indispensable to this task. Psychoanalysis, the seed of which was imported into the U.S.A. by Freud himself in 1909, was instantly recruited to this movement: analysts too could 'maximize output', and (as consultants to the advertising industry) could stimulate consumption by helping to market fetishized desires. Thus, what is distinctive about American psychiatry is the acceptance of psychoanalysis on equal terms with organic approaches (see also Chapters 1 and 5).

Kovel also discusses the failure of the post-1960 Community Mental Health movement to achieve any radically different political aims, and notes the rise of 'humanistic' psychotherapies which continue the process of psychologization – offering, for the first time on the open market, new, improved *selves*. Though several anti-psychiatric networks are currently active in the U.S.A. (e.g. the Mental Patients' Liberation Movement, and 'radical therapy'[6]), Kovel is sceptical about the potentialities of such movements; however, he concludes, 'History will out, and has its surprises'.

Peter Conrad also describes the American situation in Chapter 3, but from within a different theoretical perspective – that of medical sociology. Under the title 'On the Medicalization of Deviance and Social Control', Conrad first explains the sociological view of illness and disease as essentially constituted by cultural judgements, related to human priorities and replete with practical consequences for the person judged 'ill'. In particular, to ascribe deviant behaviour to 'illness' rather than 'badness' is to reify it (cf. Chapter 1), and to locate its significance in the individual rather than their surroundings. Conrad sees this happening on an increasing scale, as alternative forms of control become inefficient or unacceptable, and as medicine becomes 'the central restitutive agent in our society'. He takes as a paradigm case the example of 'hyperkinesis', for which almost half a million American schoolchildren receive treatment. Conrad shows how many factors determine the extent to which any particular form of deviance becomes 'medicalized' – not the least of which is the massive investment which the drug companies put into promoting the medical model.

Turning to Great Britain, Treacher and Baruch bring together the strands of recent research into the question: how did the medical profession come to dominate psychiatry? Here, a fascinating interaction can be unravelled between professional power-struggles and political changes on a national scale. One particularly significant finding is that the domination of psychiatry by medicine was established long before doctors could claim any success in treating more than a small number of disorders (notably syphilis). Treacher and Baruch also show how the supposed 'reforms' of the 1959 Mental Health Act have strengthened the medical approach; even experiments such as the 'therapeutic community' pioneered by Maxwell Jones,[7] though politically quite innocuous, have been discouraged by the removal of patients to general hospitals.

Britain has also been a centre of 'anti-psychiatry', and besides the well-known writings of Laing, Esterson and Cooper, the movement set up several organizations which attract world-wide attention in their attempts to provide true 'asylum' along the lines indicated by Laing's theories. It may seem an omission that we have not attempted to describe this work, but there are two reasons for this. One is that very good accounts are already available elsewhere.[8] The other is that this work has largely concentrated on the humane task of meeting the immediate needs of disturbed or distressed individuals; unlike, for example, Basaglia's project at Trieste (see Chapter 6), it has not attempted to return these problems – either theoretically or in practice – to the social context from which they originate. Although this work is of central importance in the field of treatment, therefore, it does not take us further in our present attempt to understand the *social* meaning of mental illness.

Next we examine developments on the continent of Europe. Sherry Turkle describes in 'French Anti-psychiatry' a situation which, although it has much in common with those already examined, contains certain unique elements. The distinctive feature of the French scene is the situation of psychoanalysis; in contrast to their American counterparts, French analysts have not been absorbed into the medical profession and, unlike virtually all English and American analysts, many are openly of left-wing political persuasion and have kept alive the subversive component of Freudianism. Sherry Turkle describes, in a discussion of the work of Jacques Lacan and of Deleuze and Guattari, the distinctive interpretation of Freud which this implies. The events of May 1968 in France represented the peak of the political ferment in France during that decade, and they had their impact in the mental health field as in every other; Sherry Turkle's chapter is particularly useful for the way in which it describes not only the attempts which have been made to re-politicize thinking about psychiatry, but also the context of events in which these attempts were made.

The events of 1968 had repercussions throughout Europe, and psychiatry was one of the instruments of authority which was frequently under attack. This period saw many short-lived attempts to overturn the rule of orthodox psychiatry, at least within the mental hospitals; in Germany, for example, the University Clinic at Heidelberg was taken over by the patients and turned into the 'Socialist Patients' Collective'. This experiment did not survive long, but the movement which it generated did; in 1975, members of it joined with others from all over the world to set up an international network concerned with alternatives to psychiatry. David Cooper[9] has recently published an account of these activities.

In Italy, although the conditions in some mental hospitals are as bad as any in Europe, remarkable experiments have been carried out in certain northern towns – where left-wing local authorities have been willing to foster progressive experiments in psychiatry. The best-known of Italy's anti-psychiatrists is Franco Basaglia, but many others have contributed to the movement for change: the towns of Parma, Reggio Emilia, Arrezzo, Ferrara and Perugia have all witnessed more or less radical transformations in their psychiatric services. Some of the doctors involved worked with Basaglia at Gorizia during the period 1962–7, when he dismantled the oppressive structure of a typically backward asylum and replaced it with something more therapeutic.[10] As he says in Chapter 6, however, the concept of a 'humane' asylum was for Basaglia a contradiction in terms, since confinement and separation were at the core of the psychiatric system of control; the opportunity to put this principle into practice came in 1971, when he was appointed to supervise the phasing-out of the Ospedale Psichiatrico in Trieste, and its replacement by decentralized community services. For Basaglia, 'mental illness' arises from the contradictions experienced by the individual in his or her social situation, and it can only be 'cured' by tackling these contradictions themselves; this, of course, is an idea shared by many theorists – but the striking achievement of Basaglia and his team is the concrete realization of this principle *in practice*. There is a resemblance between Basaglia's projects and the 'therapeutic communities' and 'community mental health services' of progressive psychiatry elsewhere in the West, but it is no more than a passing resemblance; the fundamental political aims and consequences are (as we learn in Basaglia's chapter) quite different. Like other Western nations, Italy has recently reformed legislation on mental health in order to restore in some measure the civil liberties of mental patients, and to integrate psychiatric and general medical services. In some respects, the 1978 laws reflect the influence of such work as Basaglia's; but their political impact in practice remains to be seen.

Finally we turn to Scandinavia – where ideas emanating from Europe, Britain and the U.S. have interacted with native traditions to produce, in each country, a unique but still recognizable situation. In Norway, the awareness of psychiatry's political dimension stimulated by 'anti-psychiatry' happened to coincide with heightened domestic conflict over economic policy, and this culminated in a remarkable campaign by all sections of the mental health professions against Norway's entry into the European Economic Community. (This proposal was, in fact, defeated in the 1972 referendum.) Svein Haugsgjerd, in 'Report from Norway', describes this campaign and the situation in which it arose. Despite the current hostility and suspicion among the left towards psychoanalysis, Haugsgjerd argues – endorsing the conclusions of Chapter 1 – that only such an approach can successfully articulate the relationships between mental illness and its social context. He examines two situations – the splitting up of families caused by enforced migration of labour, and the strains of mental hospital life – to show how psychoanalytic ideas can be related to social issues. Like Kovel, Haugsgjerd adopts an approach to family life, and to psychoanalytic theories about it, which is in strong contrast to the anti-psychiatric attitudes of the late 1960s (cf. David Cooper's title, *The Death of the Family*) and to some other versions of Marxism. For these authors, the family is more the victim of late capitalism than its agent, and a psychoanalytic understanding of human emotional needs is seen as essential to understanding its exploitation.

A word about the title: why 'Critical Psychiatry'?

'Psychiatry' because, unlike David Cooper's 'non-psychiatrists', the contributors to this volume all feel that mental illnesses – whatever their correct interpretation and their political significance may be – do exist, and furthermore call for specialized understanding and help. 'Critical' because we think that psychiatry should take time off from examining its patients in order to have a good look at itself, with the benefit of the insights which recent sociology and philosophy can offer. Such a self-examination will show how psychiatrists – bamboozled by their own scientific self-image – have accepted the servile position of functionaries in the modern state; emancipated from that role, hopefully they may be in a position to become critical of society itself. After all, since psychiatrists have the unenviable job of coping with the misery that accompanies our mode of social organization, they are well-placed to interpret the underlying contradictions and to diagnose the madness of our way of life. And despite its conformist image, psychiatry has absorbed into its ranks many hard-headed and courageous recruits.

This spirit of self-examination and social critique has much in common with the 'critical theory' developed by the Frankfurt School of social philosophers, who aimed to produce an understanding that would not simply reproduce society's illusions about itself. Some of what follows is directly influenced by these writings, particularly those of Jürgen Habermas.[11] This influence, however, is only one of many; and in case any should feel that our title is misleading, and somehow infringes the trade-mark of 'critical theory', I would emphasize that the term 'critical' is being used in a sense which existed long before the Frankfurt School.

Finally, it remains for me to thank the many people, too numerous to list here, who have helped to gather and to criticize the material in this book. It may be a cliché to say so, but without their copious help the book would certainly not have existed.

Notes on Contributors

David Ingleby read psychology at Cambridge University and was a Scientific Officer with the Medical Research Council for nine years, working at the Applied Psychology Unit and the Unit on Environmental Factors in Mental and Physical Illness. He currently lectures in social psychology at Cambridge, and holds a Fellowship at Darwin College.

Joel Kovel is a psychoanalyst and psychiatric educator. He is currently Associate Professor of Psychiatry, Albert Einstein College of Medicine, where he directs the residency training programme in psychiatry at the Bronx Municipal Hospital Center. He is the author of *White Rascism* (Pantheon, 1970) and *A Complete Guide to Therapy* (Penguin, 1978).

Peter Conrad is an assistant professor of sociology at Brandeis University, Waltham, Massachusetts. He is the author of numerous articles and two books on the medicalization of deviance. His books are *Identifying Hyperactive Children: The Medicalization of Deviant Behavior* (Lexington, Mass., D. C. Heath, 1976) and *From Badness to Sickness: Deviance in American Society*, co-authored with Joseph W. Schneider (St Louis, Mosby, 1980).

Andy Treacher graduated in psychology from Bristol University and then went on to complete a Ph.D. in physiological psychology at the University of Leicester. He currently teaches courses in behavioural science and clinical psychology at the University of Bristol. His primary research and clinical interests are in the area of family therapy. He trained at the Family Institute, Cardiff, and acts as a co-ordinator of family therapy at Southmead Therapeutic Day Centre.

Geoff Baruch graduated in sociology and philosophy from Bristol University in 1973. As a research student he undertook a participant observer study of a psychiatric unit in a general hospital. This project was published as a book, co-authored by Andy Treacher, entitled *Psychiatry Observed* (Routledge & Kegan Paul, 1978). He currently works as a part-time lecturer in medical sociology at University College, London. His primary research interests include the history of psychiatry, crisis intervention, and psychotherapy.

Sherry Turkle is Assistant Professor of Sociology at Massachusetts Institute of Technology. She is the author of *Psychoanalytic Politics: Freud's French Revolution* (Basic Books, 1978).

Franco Basaglia is an Italian psychiatrist and writer. His efforts to revolutionize mental health services, starting with the reform of an asylum at Gorizia (described in his book *L'istituzione negata*), and culminating in the closure of the Ospedale Psichiatrico at Trieste, have attracted world-wide attention.

Svein Haugsgjerd is a psychiatrist at the Gaustad Psychiatric Hospital in Oslo. He specializes in the psychotherapy of psychotic conditions, which he conducts both in the hospital and in private practice. He is the author of *Nytt Perspektiv pa Psykiatrien* (Pax, 1970) and has co-edited, with sociologist Fredrik Engelstad, *Seks Samtaler om Psykiatri* (Pax, 1976) and *Samspill og Endring i Familien I–II* (Pax, 1979).

1 Understanding 'Mental Illness'

David Ingleby

In this chapter I shall try to make sense of the bewildering variety of theoretical approaches which confronts anyone trying to understand the problems of psychiatry, whether as a professional helper, a seeker of help, or just an interested observer. My aim will be to show that the many conflicting viewpoints which flourish can be understood only in terms of the philosophical systems underlying them – prior beliefs about what people are, and how we should try to understand them – and that these philosophical systems are themselves based on moral or political priorities. These ideas, of course, are not new ones: they formed the main thrust of the 'anti-psychiatry' movement in the late 1960s. What I hope to show here is the deeper perspective that can be gained by seeing psychiatry in the context of the human sciences as a whole, and by utilizing recent developments in our thinking about these disciplines.

One cherished illusion which must be lost before we can hope to understand 'mental illness' is the myth which helps to keep orthodox psychiatry on the move: the belief that what we need is simply more 'findings' – that round the corner lies some vital new fact which will settle the arguments once and for all. It is this conviction which has inspired the prodigious volume of research that the past half-century has produced in an ever-increasing flow. But despite this profusion of findings, it is doubtful whether we understand matters any better now than we did fifty years ago: as Coulter[1] puts it, 'the literature on mental disorders is quite out of proportion to the adequacy of our knowledge about them'. Obviously, there is a fundamental difference of opinion somewhere about what constitutes 'adequate knowledge'; and one of the aims of this essay will be to demonstrate the error of the naïve empiricist view that knowledge simply consists in the accumulation of findings, rather like pebbles which, if stacked up in sufficient quantity, are bound to reach the sky eventually. What matters, of course, are the principles which govern the acquisition and interpretation of 'findings'; and these principles, although they are influenced by matters of fact, are not themselves discoverable empirically – they are as much *philosophical* as scientific ones.

Unfortunately, in scientific circles (and especially in psychiatry), the word 'philosophical' has come to be a term of abuse; philosophy is seen not as a liberating and enlightening activity, but as a form of primitive pre-scientific dogmatism from whose clutches we ought to be glad to have escaped. I will not deny that something called 'philosophy' did (and still does) exist deserving of these strictures; but the very chaos in which psychiatry and its related disciplines finds itself shows that science can no longer afford to lean on this as an excuse for sidestepping *all* philosophical problems. 'Psychology', in Wittgenstein's words – and he might have included psychiatry – 'contains experimental methods and conceptual confusions'; it is because researchers have cultivated *empirical* at the expense of *conceptual* sophistication that they do not realize how serious this fault really is. Get the findings in first, and the concepts will take care of themselves, says the received wisdom – reflected in the practice of regarding only fact-finding as genuine 'work', in research circles. Concepts, being 'in the mind', are supposed to have a vague and airy quality about them, so that it would not make much practical difference what form they took.

But this metaphor is totally misleading. If one is going to picture the abstract in concrete terms, then logic is actually a 'substance' infinitely harder than steel; and it follows that a science whose conceptual foundations have not been properly thought out is doomed to collapse, no matter what volume of findings is stacked up above them.

What we need, then, are not more findings – we probably have all we need, if only we knew what to do with them – but a reappraisal of the kind of explanations we should be looking for, and the kind of data which would be relevant to them. The 'great debate' in psychiatry, which professional and disciplinary lines of demarcation have so far succeeded in keeping frozen (in the English-speaking world at least), must start with the prior questions of what kind of creatures people are, and how we should go about observing and accounting for their behaviour and misbehaviour. In what follows I shall suggest that the deep structure of disagreements about psychiatry reflects an opposition of two fundamental views on these questions: one that I shall designate as 'positivist', which seeks to assimilate the human sciences as closely as possible to the natural sciences, and the other an 'interpretative' view, which sees the subject-matter and therefore the methodology of the human sciences as *sui generis*.

The reader will note that my account differs from most discussions of psychiatry, in which 'the medical model' is contrasted with non-medical alternatives: what I want to emphasize is something which criticisms of 'the medical model' often obscured – namely, the fact that classical psychiatry was basically modelled on positivism, rather than on medicine *per se*. (Indeed, it is possible to conceive of a non-positivist approach to medicine – such as von Weiszäcker's[2] 'anthropological medicine' – within which many of the objections to traditional medical psychiatry would disappear.)

These two fundamentally opposed frameworks (positivist and interpretative) are not simply conflicting theories, between which we might arbitrate on empirical grounds, simply according to which 'fits the facts' better: they correspond to what the philosopher of science Kuhn[3] calls 'paradigms' – that is, whole systems of prejudice about what constitutes useful and respectable data, what form theories should take, what sort of language scientists should use, how they should go about their business, and so on. In short, they correspond to different *mentalities*. Any observer soon realizes, too, that birds of a feather flock together in groups which reinforce their own views to the exclusion of everybody else's; to this extent, adherence to one or other paradigm is equivalent to membership of a sort of community.

This immediately raises the problem of how different mentalities can be reconciled and different communities understand each other's customs – or, in more technical terms, the 'commensurability of paradigms'. There is more than a figurative resemblance here to the problems arising when anthropologists from one culture try to understand people from another; and the most important lesson anthropology has to teach us about this problem is the need to respect the autonomy and internal coherence of the 'foreign' culture, and the impossibility of simply *invalidating* one mentality from the standpoint of another. Here is Evans-Pritchard[4] writing on Azande witchcraft:

> In this web of belief every strand depends on every other strand, and a Zande cannot get out of its meshes because it is the only world he knows. The web is not an external structure in which he is enclosed. It is the texture of his thought and he cannot think that his thought is wrong (p. 194).

And here is Professor Sir Martin Roth, founding President of Britain's Royal College of Psychiatrists, writing on psychiatry's critics:

The anti-medical critique of psychiatry represents one approach within a wider movement which has assumed international proportions and adopts a critical or derogatory stance towards psychiatry's methods, aims and social role; it is anti-medical, anti-therapeutic, anti-institutional and anti-scientific, either by expressed aim or implicitly through the dogmatic, exhortatory, diffuse and inconsistent character of its utterances.[5]

How does it come about that for Sir Martin, to criticize his profession is to abdicate both reason and humanity? One answer is suggested in Evans-Pritchard's fine phrase: 'he cannot think that his thought is wrong'.

But of course if this were the only answer, then the outlook for psychiatry – indeed, for humanity itself – would be dismal indeed. Though between any two mentalities a vast area of incommensurability exists, we possess nevertheless the means of detecting common ground and building bridges from the one to the other. If this were not so, there would be no sensible basis for choosing between different paradigms, and each would occupy its own self-contained, impenetrable world – allowing as 'admissible evidence' only that which confirms its assumptions. Despite some of the more extreme interpretations of Kuhn's views, such a relativistic conclusion is not justified in psychiatry at least: for the different contenders *do* know, to a large extent, what the others are talking about. (Some of them, such as psychiatrists turned anti-psychiatrists, have actually held at one time the positions they are opposing.) Though the different paradigms are to a striking extent self-confirming and self-contained, they could logically be brought into some relation with each other: the real issues which maintain the divisions between their holders, therefore, must lie elsewhere.

These issues are not hard to find – as I have already suggested, they are questions of values or politics. Negotiation between the holders of different paradigms is difficult, not only because each paradigm uses a different conceptual system, but because each represents different *interests*. This view, although put forward in a very sophisticated form by the social theorist Habermas,[6] is nevertheless at root a fairly straightforward one. If we wish to travel by bus, we will acquire timetables and an accurate watch, and be very alert to large red objects coming down the road; likewise, if we are concerned about the oppressive aspects of our society, we will take very seriously a theory which suggests that mental illness is a manifestation of them. Thus (although the connections between knowledge and interest which Habermas describes are a lot more complex than this), it is not difficult to grasp how different paradigms may be preferred on the basis of different values.

The traditional objection to bringing values into scientific debate is, of course, that the argument then collapses into a relativistic free-for-all which is the very antithesis of what science is supposed to be. However, Kuhn's close examination of the history of science showed that the grounds on which one paradigm is preferred to another are not exclusively scientific ones: the determinants of that choice lie to a large extent *outside* science, in social and psychological factors. (Kuhn mentioned solidarity and the pressure to conform, but solidarity is in turn based on common interests.) This view has naturally been hotly contested, since it blurs almost to vanishing-point the distinction between scientific belief-systems and (say) religious or political ones; but as Bernstein[7] has pointed out, Kuhn's conclusion is only disastrous if one presupposes, as he and most scientists traditionally have, that any choice determined by social or psychological factors is necessarily an irrational one.

Habermas, on the other hand, dismisses the view that there are only two rational modes of argument – appeal to facts, and appeal to logic – and claims that so far from knowledge being independent of moral values and human interests, it is actually 'constituted' by them. These fundamental questions of paradigm choice, therefore, are to be settled by *moral* reasoning, which is not a matter of brute force and emotion (as empiricists assumed it must be), but of negotiation and a common search for ideals. As Habermas' critics have been quick to point out, this is a difficult view to uphold unless one believes in an ultimate realm of absolute moral truths; but nevertheless it is easy to see how he reaches this conclusion, and how it offers a way of rescuing science from the relativistic chaos into which Kuhn appeared to have thrown it. The questions which the first section of this chapter will serve to open up, therefore, are: What values are enshrined in positivist psychiatry? What interests does it further, and do we want the kind of society which it leads us towards?

Our search for the 'knowledge-constitutive interests' in psychiatry is, however, hampered by the profession's own categorical insistence that there are none there; indeed, the fundamental aim of positivism, as set out by the man who gave it a name, Auguste Comte, was to resolve social problems on the basis of factual considerations alone. Those who object to 'bringing politics into science' therefore have to be shown that in the human sciences, and particularly psychiatry, politics is *already there*, just as it was in Comte's own project. My first task will be to show that the view of psychiatry as 'value-free' is pure whitewash; only when its pretensions to objectivity have been got out of the way can we proceed to discuss what, in fact, its moral premises are, and which interests it furthers.

I. The critique of positivist psychiatry

As I have stressed above, classical psychiatry was not merely an offshoot of the medical profession, springing up spontaneously in the soil of the clinic and the asylum, but was part of a much larger project in the history of man's attempts to understand himself. Positivism aimed to construct human sciences on the model of natural sciences: contemporary authorities still place psychiatry firmly within this paradigm. 'The foundations of psychiatry have to be laid on the ground of natural sciences', say Mayer-Gross, Slater and Roth.[8]

From the beginning right up to the present day, this alliance with natural science was seen as a way of lifting psychiatry above the level of particular interests and arbitrary prejudices, and giving it an impartial and detached authority. In this section, I shall try to show that what it achieves is quite the opposite.

Underlying the positivist enterprise is, of course, one major assumption: that there are no features distinguishing human beings from the rest of nature which might necessitate the adoption of a different paradigm. I shall argue that this assumption alone is such a large and implausible one as to undermine from the start any claim to impartiality: if, as the opponents of positivism have claimed, there *are* such distinctive features, then the naturalistic paradigm merely serves to distort our understanding.

I shall consider in turn the two chief elements of the paradigm: its prescriptions about how to go about collecting data, and about how to construct theories. Positivism assumes, in the first case, that observations can be made objectively – that measures can be defined operationally, and applied in a precise, replicable fashion; and in the second, that theories can be constructed on the same causal, deterministic basis as in the natural sciences. Both these fundamental principles have been challenged in their embodiments across the whole range of human sciences – from Durkheimian sociology,[9] through behaviourist psychology (Harré and Secord; [10] Gauld and Shotter[11]), to the recent criticisms of psychiatry. Although the particular objections I shall make have all been raised before by 'anti-psychiatrists', the point I want to bring out is that most of them relate not just to psychiatry, but to positivism in any form.

(A) The myth of objectivity

Perhaps the sharpest difference between positivist psychiatry and its critics arises over its concept of *data* and how to go about collecting it. The 'scientific' psychiatrist aims to collect observations on his patients in the same rigorous and detached fashion as, say, the astronomer observing stars; his critics, however, are united in regarding this as a tactic which can only obscure his vision, and render useless whatever theories (biochemical, social or otherwise) are constructed out of such data. As Laing[12] caustically put it, 'you cannot make a statistical silk purse out of a clinical sow's ear'. Anyone who has had to deal with psychiatric case-notes will recognize the style: the patient is pinned down by a few cut-and-dried epithets, with no hint of the complex ambiguities of human conduct or of the context in which the patient acts and is observed. Constantly in the background is the example provided by 'scientific' medicine: the patient reduced to a set of basic variables – temperature, pulse, blood-pressure ... emotional tone, aggressivity, reality-sense.

It is no accident that the criticisms of this ideal of objectivity in psychiatry are closely paralleled by arguments going on within psychology and sociology. The notion that social facts are 'things' which can be described like any other natural objects has been the target of continual criticism since Durkheim first articulated it in 1895. In the next section I shall say a little more about this critical tradition; the current crisis of confidence in positivist epistemology (theory of knowledge) is largely the result of work done by Wittgensteinian analytical philosophers and by the phenomenological and ethnomethodological schools of sociology. These ideas have been applied to psychiatry by Robertson,[13] Coulter[14] and Heritage; [15] their implication is that the lack of objectivity in the human sciences will never be cured simply by trying to do better – rather, it stems from the application of totally irrelevant criteria.

'Objective description' means many things. In the first place, it means that concepts should have an explicit and uniform usage, and that measurements should be *definable* in terms of the operations which give rise to them. In psychiatry, however, 'operational definition' is an obstacle in front of which whole armies of theoreticians have blunted their weapons – because, blinkered by their naturalistic assumptions, they have failed to take account of the distinctive problem of characterizing human behaviour and experience.

The root of this problem lies in the fact that the most useful descriptive concepts are simply not definable in terms of a finite set of observations; there are as many ways of expressing 'anger', for example, as there are people to get angry and situations to get angry in. None of us have much difficulty as non-scientists in recognizing anger when we see it, because we have a lifetime's experience of how the concept is applied; common sense enables us to cope with the 'open texture' of such concepts. Common sense, however, does not meet positivism's requirement of an explicit set of criteria: as the ethnomethodologist Garfinkel[16] pointed out, there are no *formal* rules according to which a reader can reconstruct, from material classified by a researcher, the precise observations on which it is based – he has to rely on a shared background of 'taken-for-granted' interpretative competence. Any attempt to specify the rules relating descriptions to situations would run into endless qualifications, special clauses, and so on; this Garfinkel dubbed 'the *etcetera* problem'. Faced with this problem, psychiatrists have responded in one of three main ways.

The first (which Clare,[17] as a sensible middle-of-the-road practitioner, adopts) is to recognize it as a problem, and to admit that 'clinical judgement' is an essential ingredient of psychiatric description; this, at least, is a realistic conclusion, but 'clinical judgement' is a blank cheque which can be filled in with any amount of tacit biases and unwritten rules, and completely undermines psychiatry's claim to be based on observations more solid than lay judgement. For the fact that clinical expertise is maintained by a professional clique is not, in itself, any guarantee of objectivity – more likely the reverse.

The second response to the 'etcetera problem' is to disguise it by offering makeshift definitions, glossing over the tacit assumptions necessary for applying them to any particular instance: most descriptions of psychiatric 'syndromes' are of this form ('flatness of affect', 'bizarre gestures', 'impulsive outbursts', 'withdrawn manner'). Of the same ilk are psychological questionnaires asking deceptively straightforward questions of the type: 'Are you usually happy?', which simply lay the onus of interpretation on the subject or the coder. (Without such interpretation, the only possible answer to such questions is, of course, 'It all depends!')

The third 'solution' is that advocated by thorough-going positivists such as Eysenck: it is to deem open-textured concepts like 'anger' or 'happiness' unsuitable for scientific purposes, and to replace 'clinical judgement' by deliberately artificial constructs such as a person's score on a test, or some physiological index such as skin conductance, blood pressure, or EEG readings. This strategy is familiar in the form of the slogan: 'Intelligence is what intelligence tests measure'; it is justified by an entirely specious analogy with 'operational definitions' in the physical sciences, in which concepts like Mass or Force are given definitions which do not correspond to everyday usage. The fallacy is, however, that the physicist's definition of 'mass' is justified by its meaningfulness and utility within a well-established theory, and the theory itself translates readily back into the language of everyday experience. None of this is true of the 'operational definitions' proposed in psychology; they are a perfect example of what Torgerson[18] and Cicourel[19] call 'measurement by fiat', and to pretend to 'validate' them by bringing them into line with the subjective judgements of psychiatrists, teachers, or whoever, is simply pulling oneself up by one's bootlaces.[20]

Of course, the psychiatrist may reply that within his province – that of 'mental illness' – these epistemological problems do not apply; what distinguishes 'symptomatology' from ordinary human conduct, he may say, is precisely that it does *not* represent the meaningful activities of human agents. He may concede that off duty, in the realm of 'normal' people, he is obliged like anyone else to make subjective, common-sense interpretations: but since (unlike most sociologists and psychologists) it is not in this realm that he operates, he may well think that he can evade Garfinkel's 'etcetera problem'.

The snag with this particular argument is that in order to *know* that he is not in the 'normal' realm, he has to make a judgement which relies even more heavily on subjective understanding than the everyday interpretations discussed above: to make a warranted ascription of insanity, he has to be sure that *none* of the ordinary ways of finding conduct intelligible actually works – and this he cannot do without applying each of them in turn, and thus invoking subjective judgement. To take a particular example, in order to categorize a patient as 'aggressive' or 'depressive', he has to be sure that they are not being *understandably* angry or sad; and to do this he must examine their behaviour in its context and apply complex cultural norms to evaluate its reasonableness. As Coulter[21] convincingly shows, this means that insanity ascriptions are inescapably rooted in common-sense cultural understanding, and to imagine that they could be grounded in something which transcends common sense (i.e. in neutral, scientific authority) simply makes no sense.

Two points have been made so far. The first is that while it may be in principle possible to state exactly the criteria for applying physical concepts, it is in principle impossible to do so for concepts describing human activities and states of mind. Descriptions of the latter are always subjective interpretations – subjective not in the sense that there *are* no criteria, but that the criteria are unstated ones, lying in the culture itself. The second point is that judgements of *insanity* are even more dependent on cultural competence, since they assert that *no* conventional interpretation can be successfully applied. The first point undermines the possibility of objective description in the human sciences generally, the second applies to psychiatry in particular.

One of the ways in which critics have sought to attack psychiatry's claim to objectivity, and supporters to defend it, is by pointing to statistics on the reliability of psychiatric diagnoses (that is, the extent to which different psychiatrists are likely to agree on the classification of cases). Published figures in fact vary widely, giving both parties ample ammunition for their case; thus, Heather[22] can conclude that 'psychiatric diagnoses are extremely unreliable', while Clare[23] claims that they are no more so than in other branches of medicine. I shall not attempt to review the relevant statistics here, because I think there are two considerations which make this issue something of a red herring.

In the first place, reliability statistics usually relate to *differential* diagnosis, i.e. to decisions about the classification of a case already presumed 'disordered' – not about whether the patient's behaviour is or is not understandable in the circumstances. The celebrated experiment of Rosenhahn,[24] in which eight perfectly sane volunteers spent several weeks in mental hospitals without their sanity being detected, suggests that such *absolute* diagnosis may be wildly inaccurate. In any case, high reliability does not necessarily indicate accuracy; Rosenhahn's study is a perfect illustration of this, since all the medical staff in the hospitals studied agreed that the volunteers were insane, but all of them were wrong! Rather, what we should be talking about is the *validity* of diagnoses – whether psychiatrists actually detect what they claim to detect; but if, as the foregoing arguments show, there is no explicit definition of precisely what it is that they are detecting, then there is no way of demonstrating publicly that they have succeeded in detecting it.

Thus, psychiatric diagnoses can never aspire to objectivity in the natural-scientific sense, and to claim that they can is merely to conceal the tacit rules, conventions and biases which necessarily govern their application. Indeed, most diagnoses forfeit their claim to be objective descriptions for the simple reason that their basic function is not a descriptive one: in everyday psychiatric practice, a diagnosis represents an administrative decision, which is governed by many other considerations besides the actual state of the patient: the family situation, the treatment available, legal considerations, and so on. This they have in common with all such 'official statistics': for sociologists, the *locus classicus* of this problem is Durkheim's[25] mistaken reliance on coroners' verdicts as an 'objective' index of suicide rates. In addition, psychiatric diagnosis may serve as an emotional defence for staff and relatives: Svein Haugsgjerd has suggested that the label 'schizophrenic' may be used to protect hospital staff against the pain of disappointment when their efforts are seen to be fruitless. Of course, not all psychiatrists are unaware of these problems (see, for example, Wing[26]); but none have convincingly demonstrated a way round them, and it would certainly come as a surprise to the rest of the human sciences if psychiatrists were to succeed where all others had failed.

Another sense in which natural sciences try to be 'objective' is in maintaining a division between subject and object; the scientist attempts, as far as possible, to eliminate the 'observer effect' or 'reactivity' produced by his intervention. But to attempt this in the study of people is quite inappropriate. Unlike the physicist, the human scientist cannot observe in a vacuum: every scientific set-up is a social situation, which the scientist cannot avoid influencing. As Laing[27] convincingly showed, the Kraepelinian method of case-presentation ignores completely the effect of the situation on the patient: to this very day, patients are paraded in front of a group of observers and described not only as if *they* weren't there, but also as if the observers weren't either. Thus, for Clare to assert[28] that the aim of this approach is to provide neutral, theory-free descriptions, and then to characterize Laing as somehow an enemy of the truth, is extraordinarily perverse.

A considerable body of recent work has shown that the same biases operate in positivist social psychology (see, e.g., Lindsay and Aronson[29]). Eysenck[30] ridiculed the idea that psychoanalysis could be (in Freud's words) 'tested on the couch', but it transpires that the sterile atmosphere of the laboratory is as replete with unknown forces as any consulting-room. The large literature on 'experimenter effects' (Rosenthal[31]) has also shown how difficult it is for the observer to avoid creating the data he needs to support his theory.

(B) The censorship of theories

The second set of presuppositions which positivism has imposed on psychiatry concerns the form which valid explanations have to take. The only legitimate mode of explanation is assumed to be *causal*, on the basis (again following Durkheim) that the laws governing human life are of the same character as those governing nature.

In psychiatry, this doctrine has what I shall call a 'strong' and a 'weak' form. The 'strong' form, variously called the 'faulty-machine' or 'disease' model, suggests that the causal factors underlying mental illness are physiological disorders; the 'weak' version still invokes causal explanation, but blames the problems on psychological or environmental factors. It has become traditional (cf. Clare[32]) to regard British psychiatry as 'eclectic' or 'non-ideological', because of its tolerance of both these points of view; but I shall show that they are simply two sides of the positivist coin, and that their dominance, so far from being inevitable, is in fact unjustified and obscurantist in its effects.

Let us take first the three sorts of evidence which are usually adduced in support of the 'organic' view, that mental illnesses have a direct physical cause. Traditionally, arguments about the *a priori* appropriateness of organic explanations are brushed aside with the retort that 'they work', so they *must* be appropriate; I shall try to show that large doses of faith are required to sustain a belief in their efficacy.

(i) *Genetic studies.* Studies of the pattern of inheritance of mental illnesses – particularly psychoses – are routinely used to bolster the claim that a genetic factor, and therefore a physical malfunction, is involved in their production. The data, however, are not as friendly to this view as they seem.

The methods by which the genetic contribution to psychiatric conditions is investigated closely parallel those used to estimate the heritability of IQ – a field in which, for some reason, arguments and criticisms have become much more sophisticated. Briefly, all the studies used as evidence for genetic transmission of 'mental illness' suffer from the same methodological weaknesses as their counterparts relating to 'intelligence'. Kamin's [33] book on IQ serves as the model for a thorough critique of this work – itself as yet unwritten, though Laing [34] and Jackson [35] have made a start. As with IQ, three sorts of data are involved.

(a) The differences in concordance rates between identical (monozygotic) and non-identical (dizygotic) twins. (The concordance rate is the probability that if one twin is affected, the other will be too.) Identical twins, of course, have all their genes in common, so that they would show a much higher degree of concordance in the case of a genetically transmitted condition: and, in many psychiatric conditions, they do. Unfortunately, this finding could come about in other ways – in the majority of studies, by biased diagnoses of zygosity of illness (because observations were not made 'blind'), and also because the *environments* of identical twins likewise have far more features in common than those of non-identical twins. The idea that identical twins are intrinsically more likely to have identity-problems, and so on, seems to be unfounded (see Clare [36]); but they do, often to a blatant extent, *identify* with each other more strongly than non-identical twins, and even though in some cases this might help the disturbed partner to remain sane, the net effect would still be to increase the rate of concordance. Then again, disturbance in one twin may make everyone more ready to 'see' disturbance in the other, which may set in motion the processes of 'deviance amplification' described by labelling theorists (see Section II) – a perfect example of a self-fulfilling hypothesis. Only if one *starts out* by rejecting all such social influences as implausible can one obtain unequivocal support for the organic model from these data.

(b) Concordance rates in separated identical twins. If these are above chance levels, then – ideally – we have a direct measure of genetic influence; conditions, however, are never in fact ideal. As in the IQ studies, samples are often biased, 'blind' diagnoses are sadly lacking, and the classification of twins as 'separated' (which is likewise seldom made 'blind') can become ludicrously flexible. [37] Furthermore, the likelihood that selective placement produces similar environments is neglected, as are age-related effects (i.e. correlations arising because twins have the same ages, and many psychiatric conditions are more likely at certain ages than at others.) Finally, no proper base rate is established from which to estimate the chance level of concordance: the circumstances surrounding such separations are never happy ones, and this fact itself may produce a higher incidence of problems in the group as a whole. All these factors combine to make the meaning of such data highly ambiguous.

(c) Incidence rates in adopted children of mental patients. Here, as with the comparisons between identical and non-identical twins, there is the possibility of environmental 'labelling'; and as with separated identical twins, there is the likelihood of selective placement, i.e. those parents who are given the children of mental patients to adopt being less able to provide a 'good' environment.

What conclusion should we then draw from these studies? According to Kamin, in the case of the data on IQ, the 'null hypothesis' that genes play no part whatsoever emerges quite unscathed; but this is a rather biased way of putting it. We could have started from the null hypothesis that genetic influences were present, but only partial; and this assumption would survive equally well. The assumption that we can understand mental illness in genetic terms alone, however, most certainly would not.

(ii) *Physiological studies.* The view that the key to mental problems could be discovered by looking inside the head was well established long before the dramatic success of the organic approach in treating syphilis (in the 1920s). As Treacher and Baruch describe in Chapter 4, 76 per cent of mental patients in the year 1890 received the privilege of an autopsy to determine the state of their brain; and in the present day, the overwhelming majority of psychiatric research is devoted to neurological or biochemical aetiology. Each new physical explanation that is put forward – defects in gross anatomy, state of arousal, serum levels, or transmitter substances – reflects faithfully the current preoccupations of neurologists.

Time and again, however, such research founders on the elementary logical problems which accompany any attempt to deduce a causal influence from a correlation. Firstly, it may be that the physiological correlate of a given mental state is a product, rather than a cause, of it – for we are generally only able to perform physiological investigations after the event. (This causal link may be very indirect, as in the conditions which are found to result from the peculiar diet of mental patients.) Secondly, both the physiological and the psychological state may be produced by another factor – for instance, by the whole complex of circumstances we call a person's 'way of life', with all its physical and psychological dimensions.

(iii) *Physical treatments.* Often it is argued that the efficacy of physical treatments (drugs, ECT, psychosurgery, etc.) is itself an indication that the original condition was physiologically determined. Two questions arise: firstly, what is the evidence for this efficacy? Many treatments only seem to be effective as long as they are believed in, either by the patient ('placebo effect'), or the medical staff ('self-fulfilling prophecy'), or both; moreover, those which are effective may only be so because of some non-physical accompaniment, e.g. the extra care or the unconscious phantasies of punishment and reparation that may accompany trips to the operating theatre. A moment's thought will reveal the practical and ethical constraints which make it very difficult for a researcher to eliminate these possibilities.

The more serious question is: what do we call 'effective'? Almost all treatments have undesirable side-effects; and if ECT reduces the pain of events only by helping the patient to forget them, or if tranquillizers make people able to handle their emotions only by leaving them with no emotions to handle, then talk of a 'cure' becomes rather ironical. In that sense, after all, death 'cures' everything.

But even if the treatment does produce a real and positive effect, what does this prove? All that actually follows is that the problem *could* have had a physical cause; not that it *did*, for it is possible for a phenomenon to arise in many different ways. Thus the value of this evidence is chiefly rhetorical: to convince the sceptic that physical causes are a *possibility*; this role we should not deny them, but anything more is plainly unwarranted.

(We could also include under this heading 'treatments' which consist of a physical intervention *producing* illness, e.g. 'psychotomimetic' drugs; provided that the treatment was not self-administered (as 'psychedelic' drugs usually are), we can rule out reversed causation, but the mechanism of causation may still be extremely indirect; and there is widespread disagreement about how closely the induced states resemble 'the real thing'.[38] The same considerations apply when we consider the similarities between certain 'functional' illnesses and the effects of brain damage or disease.)

*

An open-minded judge must conclude, I think, that all three types of evidence I have discussed have highly ambiguous implications: organic pathology is not established in the majority of psychiatric problems, nor is there any chance that it could be without attention to the problems I have listed above. But even where it is implicated, the 'faulty-machine' approach remains an inadequate one: to understand why, it is necessary to go deeper into the philosophy of explanation.

The fundamental weakness of the organic approach is that it adopts a view of causation which, despite its respectable ancestry, can be dangerously misleading. In the natural sciences, under the influence of the philosopher Hume, a 'cause' is regarded as any antecedent factor from which an event is highly predictable (always assuming that a third factor is not responsible for both). However, where the event depends on a number of factors – as in many physical sciences and most human ones – this usage can be very misleading, for it may tempt us to overlook the long and complicated pathway that leads from 'cause' to 'effect'. This is often the case when we are discussing the effect of physiological or genetic variations on human behaviour.[39] To give an extreme example, people who inherit a tall physique are very prone to bump into doorways, but the bruises on their heads are not 'caused' by their genes, even though they may be very predictable from them. Architectural fashions, urgent appointments, and lapses of attention are just as much responsible for the problem (to say nothing of the diet which enables 'genes for height' to be expressed in the first place). Thus, the outcome of any physiological state depends on many factors, some of them purely matters of social convention; to take another example, the female chromosome pair (XX) does not 'cause' a person to have a feminine personality – even though in our society the two are highly correlated – for such a personality is the product of *social* responses to a person's biological sex.

All this gives rise to what I should like to christen the 'So What?' problem in aetiology; for that is the only appropriate response to many findings which implicate physiological or genetic factors in human behaviour. A constitution which leads to one person being diagnosed as schizophrenic may, given a different life-history, be the basis of exceptional achievements; Heston,[40] in his study of the adopted children of schizophrenics, found that those who did not become psychiatric cases had more 'artistic' or 'creative' occupations than a comparison sample. Although, as I have shown above, the evidence implicating physical factors in mental illness is mostly very dubious, nobody in their right minds would deny that such influences *may* exist; the point I am trying to make here is that their discovery does not warrant the adoption of an exclusively organic approach. Thus, Siirala[41] was able to write a psychoanalytic study of communication in the families of deaf children, despite the organic origin of their defect. What matters is how a person *lives out* their physical condition.

That physical understanding by itself is inadequate is, of course, a cliché in 'eclectic' British psychiatry; but I want to show next that the narrowness of the positivist paradigm is by no means eliminated simply by introducing an alternative set of aetiological factors called 'psychological' or 'environmental'. The crucial distortions reside not in the sorts of factors that are considered causal, but in the notion of 'cause' itself. To illustrate this, I shall now consider what I called earlier the 'weak' version of positivist psychiatry.

Under this heading I am including explanations of mental illness in terms of behaviourist psychology: some positivistic renderings of psychoanalytic theory, and sociological work in the Durkheimian tradition, such as the recent study of depression by Brown and Harris.[42] 'Behaviour therapy' has sought to apply to human problems a theory of learning which barely fits the albino rat: mental illnesses are described as the result of an unfortunate history of conditioning. Psychoanalysis might be thought to start from a more sophisticated approach to mental functioning, but in practice it all too often degenerates into a sterile juxtapositioning of mysteriously inferred 'mechanisms'. The general strategy of positivist sociologists working on mental illness has been the same, but with the 'mechanisms' located outside the patient's head – in society – instead.

These approaches tend to be championed by those, such as social workers or clinical psychologists, who feel that psychiatry's defects are basically due to the stranglehold of the medical profession. I shall try to show, however, that to adopt them is to jump out of the frying-pan into another frying-pan – since they all adhere to the same paradigm of explanation as the medical model itself.

Before discussing their conception of 'causality', we should note that these approaches have inherited from the medical model the same dubious ideal of 'objectively' describing human events – only here, the problems arise not merely in describing the patient's condition, but also in characterizing the events and experiences supposed to explain it. Most environmentalist approaches start by describing the patient in much the same way that organic psychiatry does – indeed, that is hardly surprising, since they originally set out to provide 'rival' explanations. As in organic psychiatry, however, the inevitably subjective nature of such descriptions is denied, and the fact that clinical diagnoses do not merely serve to *describe* also tends to be overlooked. Even such sophisticated research as that of Brown and Harris still retains 'illness' as a descriptive category, when to do so is to beg the very question such research might be expected to answer (viz. how much of depression is *understandable?*).

When it comes to characterizing the conditions supposed to cause mental illness – be they childhood events, traumatic experiences, or social circumstances – the same misguided attempt is made to dispense with subjective meanings; here, if anything, the consequences are more serious, because it is undeniable that events affect us not for what they are, but for what they mean to us. It would seem churlish to deny that the hardships found by Brown and Harris in the environments of depressed housewives are inherently depressing – too many children, too little space, no partner, no job – but the fact is that not all are depressed by them, and in other conditions (notably wartime) these and other hardships may be associated with a dramatic *fall* in psychiatric complaints. Unless we allow that the *subjective meaning* of objective events is what influences us, we merely weaken the predictive power of environmental explanations, and leave a breach into which organic psychiatrists will eagerly step with talk of 'constitutional predispositions'. At best, most environmental research characterizes situations in terms of the meanings they *conventionally* have: thus, Coulter[43] describes the studies of 'schizophrenogenic' families which preceded Laing's as 'an attempt to scientize what amount to a set of common-sense cultural judgements'.

Thus, environmentalist approaches are even more hamstrung by natural-scientific ideals of 'objectivity' than their organic predecessors. However, more relevant to the present discussion is the fact that they rely on the same basic notion of 'cause'. In claiming that a state of mind is *determined* by a particular environment, they are in fact making a subtle claim about the nature of that mental state: for they imply that the person who has it is essentially not a rational agent. Their claims are about 'what makes people do things', rather than 'what people do'; the point is that we typically describe being *made* to do something when seeking to *excuse* behaviour for which we wish to disown responsibility. Of course, I am not trying to suggest that one can only demonstrate one's responsibility or agency by reacting to one's environment in a capricious and unpredictable way (if anything, the reverse is true); the point is that an agent's situation provides *grounds* or *reasons* for his actions, rather than *causes*. The distinction is crucial, for though human behaviour is indeed (for the most part) orderly, the 'laws' underlying it are not of the same logical type as those governing the movements of physical objects: they go hand-in-hand with agency, and in the last resort the laws themselves – unlike laws of nature – are *man-made*.

A discussion of the kinds of explanation which *are* appropriate to agents will have to wait until the second section of this chapter. The important point here is that positivist explanations essentially rule out agency; so any theorist who sets out on the quest for 'causal factors' or 'aetiology' is by no stretch of the imagination starting from a neutral or objective standpoint – he is presupposing something about the relation of conduct to its surroundings which it should be the task of research to question, not to assume. I am not, of course, arguing that people should be treated as agents *a priori*; this is a common point of view among linguistic philosophers and their disciples, but all it seems to me to accomplish is a redefinition of the word 'people'. The point is that they should not be treated *a priori* as non-agents, which is exactly what the phoney eclecticism of orthodox psychiatry tacitly achieves.

The term *reification* very usefully describes what is done when the meaningful activity of agents ('praxis') is described as if it were the outcome of an interplay of causal forces ('process'). I shall return to this concept later, but we may note here the ironical fact that self-reification is, according to the theorists we shall encounter in the next section, the very essence of mental illness: the patient ceases to experience his life as meaningful and himself as an agent, and as long as the doctor remains within the positivist framework he can do nothing but encourage this self-invalidation. As Foucault[44] puts it, the patient is 'alienated in the doctor'. Should the doctor wish to practise a therapy which stresses the recovery of intelligibility and purpose within the patient, he will abruptly discover the limitations of 'eclecticism'; for the whole of the positivist paradigm negates this aim. (Baruch and Treacher's[45] carefully documented account of psychiatry in action shows up clearly the 'double-bind' within which would-be progressive psychiatrists find themselves.) But I shall argue in a moment that this *invalidation* of the patient's experience and behaviour is what gives reification its key position in the performance of psychiatry's social role.

To sum up so far: I have claimed that the basic concepts and methods of psychiatry, so far from being neutral, in fact constitute a *paradigm*, which I have characterized as 'positivist' rather than simply medical, since it is not left behind in psychological and sociological approaches. The prescriptions of this paradigm regarding both observation and theory-construction were examined, and found to be uniquely inappropriate to its subject-matter. Psychiatry's image of itself as a science like other sciences was found to be deceptive, since (as Coulter argued) its mode of observation is not objective, but pragmatic and inherently subjective. Its mode of theorizing, while more literally borrowed from other sciences, is highly unscientific, since it begs obvious questions about the nature of the experience and behaviour it purports to explain.

This opens up an important set of questions. As long as we accepted the view of psychiatry's supporters, that its aim was to seek the truth in the only rational way available, then we could not attempt to understand it in terms of other values and interests – just as the pre-Kuhnian view of science (put forward by such philosophers as Karl Popper) ruled out of court any considerations of sociology or politics in scientific activity. If, however, psychiatry *does* contain presuppositions in Kuhn's sense, then we may ask what influenced the choice of these particular ones. All my preceding arguments, then, have been necessary to open up the question we shall now consider.

Why positivism?

Why should psychiatry, from the very beginning, have sought to pattern itself on the model of the natural sciences? Kuhn would probably answer this question in terms of conformity and persuasion: psychiatrists identified with the medical profession, and could not afford to isolate themselves from it by challenging its positivist assumptions – and medicine, in turn, could not alienate intellectual orthodoxy by denying the primacy of science. To invoke 'conformity', however, merely moves the question one stage further back: for why was the medical profession psychiatry's reference-group, and why did natural sciences enjoy their primacy? The answer to this, I believe, can only come from an examination of psychiatry's history and function as a social institution. It is this which determines the practice of psychiatrists, while theory merely provides an elaboration and rationalization of it. Thus, I shall argue that positivist models not only generate techniques through which the psychiatrist can carry out his socially ordained function, but provide an essential smokescreen behind which the real nature of that function is concealed.

The social function of psychiatry can be summed up as the control of deviance; that is, the norms of mental 'health' and 'illness' are essentially matters of cultural judgement, although positivism misrepresents them as matters of empirical fact. It is probably Thomas Szasz[46] who has done most to denounce publicly the claim that psychiatry is 'value-free'. Szasz's analysis, however, suffers from too simple a picture of the norms against which the mental patient is deviating: 'madness' is not the same as 'badness', since it violates at a much more basic level the conventions governing thought and social relationships. What the 'mad' person is up to does not (ostensibly, at any rate) have a place in the everyday vocabulary of motives – a fact which led Lemert[47] to describe it as 'residual' deviance.

Probably the most accurate and useful account of the meaning of insanity is that offered by Coulter, whose social philosophy enables him – unlike Szasz – to see rationality *itself* as basically a moral concept, and 'cognition as a moral order'.[48] However, that same philosophy also prevents Coulter from making any kind of critique of this moral order, and of psychiatry's role in maintaining it; for him, it is 'not intelligibly subject to doubt'. He thus follows the tenets of linguistic philosophy and ethnomethodology to their logical conclusion: a relativism which maintains that rationality, and the nature of social activities, can only be what people say they are. Thus Coulter's analysis, though unsurpassed as a *description* of psychiatric practice, comes to a full stop at the very point from which I want to take off.

We may wish therefore to go back to Szasz, who *does* allow himself to criticize both prevailing conceptions of normality and the role of psychiatry; but his efforts are undermined again by simple-minded preconceptions. Szasz's moral ideal is personal liberty (in the negative sense of 'freedom from constraint', rather than 'being enabled to act'); psychiatrists are enemies of liberty because they seek to impose a 'collectivist' society, in which the needs of the group are set above those of the individual. As Sayers[49] trenchantly shows, Szasz's philosophy is none other than our old friend from the nineteenth century, laissez-faire individualism – the ideology of 'free enterprise'; it is, of course, impossible to set the needs of *all* individuals above those of society as a whole, and the opposition between individual and society which this implies is logically absurd. Individualism and collectivism can never be genuine alternatives, and conflict has to be analysed, not in terms of abstract entities like 'individual' and 'society', but in terms of particular interested parties: this the anti-Marxist Szasz is not prepared to do, so that his analysis of the politics of psychiatry comes to a dead end.

Thus, Szasz is correct in his insistence that psychiatry is concerned with 'problems of living', not with the maintenance of some criterion of health lying outside morality and culture; but the conflicts which give rise to these 'problems of living' do not stem from a contradiction between the abstractions 'individual' and 'society', but from the tension between human needs and demands and the *particular* social institutions (work, the family, education, 'politics') which are supposed to provide for them. My analysis[50] – for which I claim no originality – starts from the premise that these institutions in their present form do not represent 'the common good', but a particular set of interests which conceal themselves behind the notion of 'economic progress'. Psychiatry, in turn, protects the efficient functioning of these institutions by converting the conflict and suffering that arises within them into 'symptoms' of essentially individual (or at best familial) 'malfunctioning'; it thus attempts to provide short-term technological solutions to what are at root political problems.

The foundations of such an analysis were laid by Michel Foucault in his influential work, *Madness and Civilisation*.[51] The task which medical psychiatry inherited in the nineteenth century was that of confining civilization's misfits in a place where they could not disturb the smooth harmonious surface of social life, the chief offenders being, as Foucault shows, the 'idle poor'. But while Foucault's analysis still has relevance today – witness the work of Franco Basaglia described in Chapter 6 – I believe a considerable modification of his views is necessary to take into account two important changes which the medical model has led to. These are, firstly, the 'psychiatrization' of the whole population – whereby mental illness is not seen as confined to a particular segment of humanity, but as potentially occupying segments of *everybody's* mind. Whereas previously one was either mad or sane, mental disorder is now seen as an illness which, like influenza or lumbago, can be *partial* and *temporary*. Secondly, as a necessary part of the same process, the feat of segregating mental suffering and conflict apart from 'normal' life is achieved not by brute force, but by ideas: for iron bars and chains are rendered unnecessary if the medical ideology can successfully *define* the patient's condition as lying outside the realm of meaningful human experience.

It is here that the distinctive role of positivism emerges for, as we saw above, its whole effect is to translate what it deals with from the human order into the non-human – what I called 'reification'. As long as a person's actions are seen as praxis, they tend to be taken seriously – even if being taken seriously, at times, leads to the agent being bumped off. But process – the blind workings of nature – evinces no such respect: it does not need to be argued with or fought against, but can be manipulated in whatever way suits the manipulator – and if it is defined as a 'pathological' process, then nobody in their right mind can deny that it ought to be got rid of. Hence we see the enormous potential of medicine as an instrument of social control – a potential which is not confined to the field of psychiatry (see Illich[52]; Waitzkin and Waterman;[53] Baruch and Treacher[54]). Moreover, although what I called above the 'strong' form of positivism (the 'faulty-machine' model) is the ideal way of removing all blame from social institutions, the environmentalist version is hardly more threatening to the *status quo*: for it too denies that the patient's response to his or her surroundings is intelligible and *valid*.

Thus we see that the inappropriateness of the positivist paradigm, in rational terms, is precisely what makes it so appropriate to the task of preserving existing institutions from the threat of change. Psychiatry takes on itself the responsibility for people's pain and frustration; it confiscates their problems, redefines them as 'illnesses', and (with luck) exterminates the symptoms. Come unto me, all ye who labour and are heavy laden (it says), and I will give you – oblivion. As this apparatus perfects itself, so the goal of a society truly fit for human habitation recedes further and further into the future. Radical politics, and the undermining of psychiatry, are thus inseparable from each other; moreover, dismantling the enormous mystification of social life which psychiatry has built up over the last hundred years is not a task to be completed overnight. In the next section we shall examine the progress that has been made towards this goal.

II. Interpretative approaches to psychiatry

As we saw in the first section, many who have sought to escape from the paradigm adhered to by traditional psychiatry have fallen short of their goal, and ended up merely by embracing a different (psychological or sociological) version of positivism. Indeed, the hegemony which natural-scientific ideas have enjoyed over the last hundred years has made it hard to do otherwise, since it has become virtually taken for granted that there *are* no other valid forms of knowledge. Consequently the approaches we shall examine in this section are less popular, respectable and academically established than the positivism they set out to replace. Positivists themselves have regarded these approaches with a mixture of contempt and bewilderment – for, in the words of Evans-Pritchard, 'they cannot think their thought is wrong'.

In subsuming these alternatives under a single paradigm I am, of course, doing violence to some important distinctions; and there are many authors who, because of their torn loyalties, hover uncertainly between one paradigm and the other. Nevertheless we may define the essence of the alternative paradigm simply by standing the presuppositions of positivism on their head.

Thus, contrary to positivism's 'naturalistic' assumption, that there are no features distinguishing human from natural reality which might necessitate the adoption of a different paradigm, the writers in this section assume that there *are* such features. The crucial difference ascribed to human beings (not a unique property, perhaps, but one which emerges gradually in higher animals) is the capacity for meaningful behaviour or 'praxis' – the ability to intend or express; furthermore, the nature of praxis is such that it cannot be either described or explained as if it were (as Durkheim thought) a 'thing'. In the first place, praxis cannot be *described* 'objectively', since exhaustive operational definitions of the procedures used to classify it are beyond our reach; and secondly, meaningful conduct has to be *explained* not in terms of its causes, but in terms of the agent's intentions, motives, reasons, grounds, etc. Most important of all, once we abandon positivism the very distinction between describing and explaining ceases to be hard and fast, since the two processes are combined in the single act of *interpretation*. Since this act has such a central place, I propose to call the alternative paradigm 'interpretative'.

The various approaches which can be subsumed under this heading differ mainly in their view of the act of 'interpretation'. A full history of this concept would be out of place here, and in any case beyond my means, but its ancestry is a long one. Aristotle's 'dialectical' (as opposed to 'physical') explanation implies a version of it; so too does the nineteenth-century German distinction between *Geisteswissenschaften* and *Naturwissenschaften*. 'Historical' explanation,[1] and Dilthey's hermeneutics, are other versions, along with Husserl's phenomenology, Weber's *Verstehen*, and Schutz's synthesis of the two. The Chicago-based school of Symbolic Interactionism, like English analytic philosophy, also treats in depth the problems of interpretation, and these together with Schutz's social phenomenology all influenced ethnomethodology, with its concept of 'accounting' for behaviour.[2] Freudian psychoanalysis combines interpretative methods with some of the tenets of positivism – a paradox which, I shall argue below, is not the result merely of torn loyalties, but of a unique way of looking at people. Apart from psychoanalysts, our list is made up mainly of philosophers and sociologists; with the exception of phenomenologists such as Merleau-Ponty or Jaspers, psychologists have habitually treated interpretative approaches with disdain (though there are currently signs of a shift in attitudes).

My catalogue makes 'interpretation' sound a very specialized, not to say academic, activity; but this impression is seriously misleading. For interpretative approaches, in contrast to positivism, start from very basic forms of understanding – judgements we make about each other from the moment when, as children, we grasp the difference between people and things. Interpretation is something we do all the time, even if (like M. Jourdain speaking prose) we do not realize it; so it is easier for a Laing or a Goffman to gain a popular readership than it is for a Kallmann or a Kraepelin, because their conceptual world is at root a familiar one.

Some interpretative approaches, however, stay closer to common sense than others, and along this continuum lies an important difference in outlook, which I will use as a basis for organizing the material in this section. Ethnomethodology, symbolic interactionism, phenomenology and analytic philosophy all tend to give accounts of what a person is up to in terms of what he – or his fellows – *thinks* he is up to; some of these writers even deny the validity of any other terms. On the other hand, both Marxism and psychoanalysis argue the need for what Habermas calls 'depth hermeneutics': interpretations which actively criticize and transcend people's own understanding of themselves. We can see already how different interests will, as Habermas describes, inform these two approaches to interpretation; the former being concerned to improve understanding of another person's point of view ('practical' interest), the latter to challenge their assumptions and thereby increase their degree of autonomy ('emancipatory' interest).

As applied to the problems of psychiatry, the first of these approaches may be termed 'normalizing'; [3] it starts from the assumption that common sense (or some elaborated version of it) is capable of doing justice not only to ordinary behaviour, but also to that of mental patients. ('Anti-psychiatry' usually incorporates some such point of view.) We will consider this position in detail first.

'Normalizing' approaches

I have organized the material under this heading according to the particular factor by which it seeks to make behaviour intelligible. Common-sense understanding generally tries to make sense of actions by invoking three sorts of factors: their *context*, their *purpose*, and the *code* of conventions that structures them; and this three-way division provides a useful set of pegs on which to hang the various 'normalizing' approaches. Of course, it will become apparent as we go along that every interpretation necessarily invokes all three factors; the differences are therefore merely a matter of emphasis.

(i) *Contextual approaches*. Stripped of its context – as it usually is in positivist psychiatry – no behaviour makes sense; many attempts to 'normalize' so-called mental illness have therefore sought to bring back this vital information by considering the patient's family, the wider social situation, and the medical encounter itself. Such studies implicitly claim that *anybody* experiencing such situations might react in the same way. By this is meant not that the situation would probably cause illness in anybody (which is simply the 'environmentalist' version of positivism), but that in relation to its context, the so-called illness is in fact perfectly intelligible behaviour.

Family contexts have most often been studied in connection with schizophrenia; the psychoanalytic theory of neurosis is, of course, based on early childhood experiences, but in a rather more indirect way which we shall examine later. Of the studies of schizophrenics' families, the well-known volume *Sanity, Madness and the Family* by Laing and Esterson [4] is practically the only methodologically aware application of an interpretative approach; while there are numerous other studies, almost all are 'interpretative by default' – that is, they are full of subjective interpretations, but because they are so concerned to deny the fact, they never permit the reader to see who is making the interpretations and on what basis. To say this, however, is not to deny that Laing and Esterson drew heavily for their inspiration on the work of positivists such as the Palo Alto school (Bateson, Haley, Jackson, *et al*.), Lidz, and Wynne.[5]

In the Preface to the second edition of their book, Laing and Esterson state their claim: that 'the experience and behaviour of schizophrenics is much more socially intelligible than has come to be supposed by most psychiatrists'. (It is, of course, irrelevant to object as Clare[6] does that the authors are not entitled to talk about 'schizophrenics' if they do not believe in the reality of the illness – there is nothing to prevent us today talking about witches, even if we do not believe in the Devil.) The authors call their approach 'existential phenomenology', but it could perhaps better be described as a mixture of common-sense understanding and applied linguistic philosophy; their approach actually differs from the phenomenology of Jaspers, Binswanger, and the early Laing,[7] in that they do not attribute to the patients a unique way of experiencing their situation. Rather, what warranted these patients' withdrawn, suspicious and hostile behaviour was said to be the 'untenable situation' they occupied within their suffocating and oppressive families; if they seemed paranoid, it was because people really were out to get them. Any more subjective disturbance, of the kind previously characterized by Laing as 'ontological insecurity', revealed itself as something located not in the patient but in the 'language-games' played by the family as a whole. According to Pateman,[8] 'what these patients need is not a therapist but an epistemologist'; just as rationality, according to Wittgenstein, has its grounds not in the individual but in the social communication system as a whole, so too may its opposite, 'thought disorder'. The patients are 'mystified', because they cannot learn within their family a logical way of talking, and thereby thinking, about their experience in the family (cf. also Habermas' concept of 'distorted communication'[9]).

Sanity, Madness and the Family does not provide a formal theory linking the observed features of family life to the schizophrenic's 'symptoms'; like a novel in this respect, it relies instead on the unformalizable interpretative skills of the intelligent and humane reader to bridge this gap. To have expected the authors to provide such a formal theory would be asking them to adopt a paradigm which they deliberately and advisedly rejected. In addition, provided one accepts the authors' account of their sampling method, it is misguided to complain, as does Wing,[10] of the lack of 'normal' controls: for the hypothesis of social intelligibility is not to be confused with that of environmental causation. The other often-repeated criticism, that the patients in this book are not 'really' schizophrenic, rebounds damagingly on the critics – for if eleven out of eleven randomly chosen diagnoses of schizophrenia are incorrect, the overall rate of misdiagnosis must be getting on for 100 per cent. And if psychiatrists fail to recognize the cases in this book as typical, it merely betrays how unsympathetically and superficially they are in the habit of perceiving their own patients.

Laing and Esterson, of course, simply remove the problem one stage further back: what is the context of this crazy family situation itself? What emotional needs do these patterns of distorted communication serve, and how do they fit into the culture as a whole?

The emotional dynamics of 'distorted' family relationships have been studied largely in psychoanalytic terms, e.g. by Esterson[11] (who investigated in depth one of the cases from *Sanity, Madness and the Family*), Mannoni[12] and Stierlin;[13] the projection, expelling, scapegoating and double-binding that occur in the 'schizophrenic' family are seen as supporting the psychological defences of individual family members – to such an extent that the consequences of abolishing them can be as disastrous as the original problem.

Such accounts, of course, tend to reduce family disorders back into the language of individual psychology, while what is much more important – and much less well understood – is the relationship between both family and individual dynamics and *society as a whole*. Although *Sanity, Madness and the Family* went as far as was logically necessary to achieve its stated aim, it came as a disappointment to many readers that Laing never went beyond the level of the family in his attempt to relate 'madness' to its social context – or even when he did, that he expressed his diagnosis in vague and ahistorical terms (see Deleuze and Guattari[14] and Jacoby[15]). Joan Busfield[16] has made a solitary attempt to understand the 'double-binds' experienced by the adolescent in family life, in terms of contradictory values built into our society itself; otherwise, the only relevant writings seem to be those of the 'Freudian Marxists' discussed in my next section.

Study of the family context, however, may mislead not only by suggesting that the family exists in a vacuum, but also by ignoring the many other institutions which comprise a person's social context. The assumption that only home life has emotional significance does, in fact, reflect a sort of half-truth: for, as Joel Kovel points out in Chapter 3, the modern family has had to carry the full burden of emotional involvements withdrawn from the community, as the latter fractures and falls apart under the impact of the economic forces of advanced capitalism. Certainly, most people experience only their 'private' lives in human terms; but psychotherapists who, in their preoccupation with the family, also forget the maddening aspects of the wider society are merely colluding with those economic forces and producing ideology, not science.

Most studies of 'mental illness' in its wider social context come from the environmentalist offshoot of positivism; like the corresponding family studies, they are interpretative only by default. Worse still, they often rely on crude epidemiological data such as hospital admission rates; as we saw above, such information reflects people's mental states very indirectly, if at all. This means that most cross-cultural statistics are virtually useless, because such factors as diagnostic practice and the availability of psychiatric services vary widely between cultures. The same considerations apply to studies of the relationship between mental illness and social class, since these are virtually cross-cultural studies too; although most researchers report a strong association between poverty and (e.g.) hospital admission rates, it is very hard to know what this association means. Do these statistics tell us something about the problems which unemployed or overworked, underpaid, poorly housed and ill-nourished people actually have, or about the way society processes their complaints? Most researchers interpret the connection between economic hardship and mental illness in terms of an intervening variable called 'stress', but this term adds little to the explanation. If 'stress' is *inherent* in certain situations, then it is a redundant concept; while if (as is much more likely) it is a function of the *meaning* which the situations hold for their occupants, then we need a theory of 'subjective meanings', and this is precisely what no positivist psychology can offer. Postulating variables like 'stress' is no substitute for a properly interpretative account of the way people's situations, as they perceive them, give them grounds for their conduct. At the level of class or nation, such studies are rare indeed: I would mention here Franz Fanon's[17] account of the vicissitudes of colonial life, and Sennett and Cobb's study[18] *The Hidden Injuries of Class*, which focuses on the American blue-collar worker's situation. The 'Freudian Marxists' discussed later also offer their own distinctive analysis of the relations between culture and psycho-pathology.

Understanding people's 'symptoms' in terms of their social situation is perhaps easier when we define the latter in more specific terms. Here I am returning to the idea put forward in Section I, that 'mental illness' is an intelligible response to conflict between people's needs and the demands (or constraints) placed on them by their particular social roles. Although in positivistic studies of the social environment, both 'cause' and 'effect' and the link between them are defined in such a way as to *conceal* any such intelligibility, it can be instructive to take as a starting-point the positivists' discovery that certain roles are associated with particular patterns of 'symptomatology'. I shall consider four examples of this.

The first case is one we have already considered under the heading of family studies. The diagnosis of 'schizophrenia' tends often to be made in adolescence, i.e. during the transition from juvenile to adult roles; as we saw above, Laing and Esterson sought to demonstrate the intelligibility of such 'symptoms' when seen against a background of contradictory family demands, and these demands were in turn interpreted by Busfield as reflecting contradictions endemic to the adolescent's role. But although the young schizophrenic became the *cause célèbre* of anti-psychiatry, I believe that this was to the detriment of the movement as a whole: the depressed housewife, the senile psychotic, and the maladjusted schoolchild do not lend themselves so readily to the part of culture-hero – nor, in general, can they afford the fees of an existential psychoanalyst – but they are far more representative of psychiatric cases. Moreover, as I shall try to indicate briefly below, they illustrate somewhat more graphically the relationship between roles and 'symptoms'.

To start with, the high incidence of depression among housewives is a 'symptom' that the women's movement has been quick to decode. Brown and Harris[19] have estimated its prevalence in a London sample of working-class women at 23 per cent, and have shown that having small children, no outside employment, no stable partner, and poor housing, can render it endemic. From the feminist point of view, it is somewhat perverse to speak of 'illness' at all here: one might more readily imagine that there was something odd about women who were *not* made miserable by such burdens. This brings out very clearly the fact that deciding what constitutes a 'warrantable' response to one's situation is largely and unavoidably a political decision. The work of Brown and Harris, therefore, goes a long way towards demolishing its own positivist presuppositions.

One group without a 'liberation movement' to voice their predicament is the elderly, who again show a characteristic pattern of mental illness; nevertheless, Robert Kastenbaum[20] has maintained a solitary but determined argument that the indignities and deprivations of the role which our society allocates to its members, as soon as they cease to be useful to the labour-market, are quite sufficient to warrant the anger, despair and confusion which psychiatrists routinely diagnose as 'senile psychosis' and so on.

Children, of course, form the other obvious group which lacks organized representation of their political interests. As I have tried to show in an earlier paper,[21] child psychology in general tends to be heavily biased against the child; more specifically, Conrad (Chapter 3) shows how the currently fashionable diagnosis of 'hyperkinesis' reifies and invalidates the rebellious actions whereby schoolchildren express their boredom and frustration with their allotted roles. When hyperkinesis becomes an 'epidemic', as it has in the U.S.A., we should perhaps cease talking about maladjusted children, and think instead about the maladjustment of their schools and families.

Other examples could be added to this list. Maucorps[22] discussed the 'social vacuum' responsible for many apparently bizarre symptoms in demoralized and depopulated rural areas. Haugsgjerd (Chapter 7) considers the consequences in psychological terms of the changed way of life which is forced on sectors of the Norwegian population by 'economic forces' – that is, the interests of capital. Jules Henry,[23] in *Culture against Man*, anticipated many of the analyses I have mentioned of Western family life, schooling and ageing. Despite all these examples, however, such work is yet in its infancy: I have not mentioned at all the vicissitudes of two important roles – being employed, and being unemployed.

Such research is unlikely to develop under the aegis of orthodox psychiatry, which quite literally has no use for it – since its mandate is not to change society, but individuals. True, it was a constant theme of Freud's writings that mental illness arises from the conflicts and tensions of social life; but while he argued that the constraints giving rise to repression and neurosis were intrinsic to civilization itself, the view which we represent in this book sees these constraints (e.g. family and work roles) as social conventions, tied up with the maintenance of a particular economic system, and changeable if – and only if – that system can be changed.

Some orthodox psychiatrists, even though they may reject psycho-analysis, also see mental illness as arising from the 'stress' of living without certain basic human needs and comforts. Like Freud, how-ever, these environmentalists fail to see that human needs are (to some extent, at least) a social construction: very few 'life-events' (to use the jargon of this school) have a fixed, determinate effect – their impact depends on the *meaning* ascribed to them, and this meaning is a social variable. Thus, the reason why a situation which is today experienced as oppressive may not have been so regarded a hundred years ago is that we have different expectations of life; as Kovel reminds us, capitalism itself helped to nurture precisely those needs for 'self-realization' and 'autonomy' which at the same time it thwarts. Women today would perhaps not find their situations so depressing if they had not come to regard themselves as human beings: old people would not miss love if they had not once been obliged to attach such a value to it. The 'human nature' being thwarted is largely *second* nature, so it becomes impossible to describe one pole of the contradic-tions as 'inner' and the other as 'outer'.

The psychiatric context. As well as showing how psychiatric dis-turbance may arise as an intelligible response to social conditions, the 'normalizing' approach also has a lot to say about society's response to the disturbance – that is, about the institution of psychiatry itself. Although this work has mostly centred on the tangible, bricks-and-mortar institution of the mental hospital, it is important to remember that the concept includes something wider – the practice of psychia-try, whether or not it takes place in a mental hospital; and to the way psychiatric ideas are incorporated within 'common sense' itself. For as the mental hospitals are phased out, more and more treatment takes place in the doctor's surgery and the general hospital; but the mental patient is still just as effectively incarcerated within his role. Moreover, this role is internalized within the patient's own thinking and that of the people around him or her, and it guides everybody's self-interpretations, whether or not they ever become patients.

Nevertheless, it is within the mental hospital situation that the medical encounter can be most closely examined. The classic studies here are those of Erving Goffman; drawing on the sociological tradition of Symbolic Interactionism, Goffman applied the concepts of 'total institution', 'degradation ceremony', and 'moral career' to the asylum situation,[24] and described in grim and compelling detail the *cognitive*, rather than simply physical, pressures which kept the patient in their place. (It was these pressures which Rosenhahn's[25] volunteers experienced at first hand.) Of course, it was known even to positivists (e.g. Wing and Brown[26]) that the traditional mental hospital was not a particularly good place to get 'better' in.

The institution of psychiatry was also studied, in a way that transcended the hospital situation itself, within the framework of 'labelling theory'. Scheff[27] argued, following the work of Balint[28] and others on medicine's 'normal cases', that psychiatric illnesses were socially constructed, just as physical ones were; they represented schemas according to which people organized and interpreted their own and other people's 'sick' behaviour. Scheff claimed, moreover, that the states supposedly characteristic of 'mental illness' were actually very widespread in the normal population (cf. Pasamanick[29]); if a person was not *labelled* sick, these states were overlooked, but if he was, they provided further 'proof' that the diagnosis was correct. Thus, the diagnosis of mental illness represented a point of no return; as Lemert[30] and Becker[31] had argued in their general theories of deviance, society provided a kind of positive feedback which resulted in 'deviance amplification', as the patient internalized other people's judgements of him. ('Deviance amplification' in the opposite direction is illustrated in the famous study by Rosenthal and Jacobson,[32] who found that children's cognitive performance was improved by telling their teachers that they were 'bright'.) The work of labelling theorists added depth to Goffman's concept of mental illness as a 'career', which many psychiatrists must have taken as just a bad joke.

These studies of the mental patient's role may help to make intelligible many aspects of his or her conduct after being diagnosed; but they do not, of course, leave us any wiser about the psychiatrist's conduct. For Goffman, psychiatry is simply *there*; as we saw in Section I, Szasz's attempts to explain what it is *doing* there lack cogency, and the theory which this book sets out to promote (see Chapters 2 and 4) is still very much in its infancy. But what I hope has been learned in this section is that what one thinks psychiatrists are up to depends crucially on what one thinks their patients are up to; and the latter question cannot be answered without taking an essentially political stand on what constitutes a 'reasonable' response to a social situation.

Thus, no amount of purely empirical data will enable us to decide whether to take sides with orthodox psychiatry or its critics; and this, as Hesse[33] argues – following Habermas – may be an unavoidable feature of any social theory.

(ii) *Redefinition of goals.* The second tactic in the 'normalizing' approach is to ascribe an unrecognized *purpose* to the behaviour in question. Of course, this goes hand in hand with the presentation of the context of action (as well as the assumption of a code), so that no studies can be said to fall into this category alone; but two key ideas in anti-psychiatry centre chiefly on the question of purposes. The first is the idea that the 'sick' behaviour is a form of protest; the second, that it is a kind of self-cure.

The 'symptom as protest' school finds its strongest support in Goffman's studies of asylum politics. 'If you rob people of all customary means of expressing anger and alienation and put them in a situation where they have never had better reason for having these emotions, the natural recourse will be to seize on what remains – situational improprieties.'[34] Outside the asylum, this view is implicit in (for example) Laing and Esterson's family studies; in the feminist interpretation of housewives' depressions; and in Conrad's views on 'hyperkinetic' schoolchildren. The idea gains a deeper perspective within the thinking of Sartre and Marcuse, in which the 'dregs' of the capitalist system – the deviants and drop-outs – constitute, in Hegelian terms, the 'determinate negation' of that system; hence the idea mentioned above, of 'the schizophrenic as culture-hero'. According to David Cooper,[35] 'all delusions are political declarations and all madmen are political dissidents'.

Perhaps because it was so inadequately formulated, however, this idea became the weakest plank in the anti-psychiatric platform. It was in fact the Left who attacked it most strongly: Sedgwick,[36] Mitchell,[37] Gleiss[38] and Jacoby,[39] all objected that this 'romanticizing' of society's victims distracted attention from the real need for coherent, rational political action – and didn't help *them*, either. Unfortunately, these critics reverted to an astonishingly positivistic 'us/them' model of mental illness; the real point, surely, is not that psychiatric problems lack political significance, but that they are not *effective* forms of social action.

For the 'symptom as protest' view glosses over the differences between the kinds of behaviour that psychiatrists deal with, and conscious, socially intelligible and potentially effective forms of protest.

In Morel's original case of 'dementia praecox',[40] there was perhaps not much difference – the boy's chief 'symptom', apparently, consisted of hatred of his father! – but most people, after all, refer themselves for treatment, and do so precisely because they do not understand what is going on. Yet rather than revert to the orthodox view of illness, as the Left has been inclined to do, what seems called for is a concept of interpretation more subtle than the common-sensical 'normalizing' approach can offer: and this will be the topic of our final section.

The concept of 'symptom as self-cure' has similar shortcomings. Laing's suggestion that 'catatonic' withdrawal represents a form of meditation has an appealing simplicity; and his idea of psychosis as a 'voyage into inner space', 'an attempt to overcome our normal state of appalling alienation', is a popular one by now. Indeed, the basic idea is not all that original: Freud himself spoke of psychotic patients 'attempting to cure themselves by becoming hysterical',[41] and the concept of controlled therapeutic regression is well established in psychoanalysis today. The key word, however, in these quotations is 'attempt'; Freud certainly did not imagine they would *succeed*, and Laing offers little evidence that they do (though to be fair, the societal reaction to psychosis is so destructive that it is hard to imagine the idea ever receiving a proper test). If such symptoms are attempts at self-cure, they are neither deliberate nor effective ones; just as the psychotic 'protest' plays straight into the hands of the oppressors by inviting its own invalidation, so the 'cure' perpetuates the state of alienation by merely expressing it in a more colourful and intransigent form.

(iii) *The concept of 'code'*. In appealing to a special 'code', the normalizing approach is claiming that the problem behaviour does not have the superficial meaning which we ascribe to it, but instead belongs within a framework which accords it quite a different meaning. Such a framework is really a form of symbolic *environment*, which merely shows the weakness of my classification: for this category is really an extension of the contextual approach, and the studies of schizophrenics' families as well as Goffman's asylum ethnography belong here as well.

The subcultural theory of deviance put forward by Becker[42] and others suggests that much conduct is regarded as 'sick' simply because 'straight' observers do not understand the meaning that it has in its own subculture. This idea has obvious relevance in the case of diagnoses of mental illness made by professionals to whom the patient's culture is an alien one. For example, it has been found that West Indian immigrants are commonly seen as 'aggressive' by English welfare officials on the basis of their intonation patterns, which have been superimposed on to English from African languages. Among the same group, the relatively frequent diagnoses of 'psychosis' may be due in part to English psychiatrists not appreciating that trance states, spirit possession and the like can be part of a normal life-style.

Not many problems in psychiatry, however, are likely to be amenable to solutions of this sort, where the code invoked is of a recognized and public kind. The 'decoding' of most symptoms calls for a rather different kind of methodology, which goes beyond the limits of common sense; the psychoanalytic approach, which alone has attempted this, invokes a 'code' which we fail to recognize, not because it belongs to a foreign culture, but because it is a part of our own mentality too close for comfort. This, however, is to anticipate our next section.

Having outlined the essentials of the 'normalizing' approach, we may now ask: how does it compare with positivism, and how successfully does it deal with the phenomena of psychiatry?

Clearly, the positivist ideals of 'objectivity' are not met by this form of interpretation, and indeed its exponents would claim that they never could be in any human or scientific 'human science'. Its concepts are not operationally definable, its observations cannot be literally reconstructed, and the observer cannot pretend not to influence the situation he observes. The positivist will deplore the fact that such work draws so heavily on taken-for-granted resources of judgement and interpretation though, as we have seen, his paradigm also leans on these – while no one is looking. In addition, interpretative theories do not take the form of rigid laws of causation, but specify instead configurations of context, motive and code which make actions intelligible; in few situations could anything like a *prediction* be made, for the uniqueness of persons and situations is implicit in this approach. Hence, such theories do not generate an easily reproducible technology of behavioural research and intervention of the kind that positivism – falsely – promised. Moreover, to the extent that they identify certain issues as moral rather than factual questions (e.g. whether the depressed housewife is really 'ill'), they do not claim to be value-free.

To the positivist, then (in Haugsgjerd's words), such approaches represent 'a tide of obscurantism', while to psychotherapists and the like, terms such as 'hermeneutic' suggest 'a promise that one day their kind of work will get its fair share of scientific glory'. The appeal of such theories, once the vain hope of emulating 'hard' science is renounced, lies in their refusal to deny the differences which we all know to exist between people and things. In consequence of this refusal, reification and individualism – the inevitable accompaniments of positivism – can be avoided: the pseudo-technological, ideological interest becomes replaced by the 'humanistic' one of understanding other people's points of view. Moreover, the fact that only qualified psychiatrists could apply positivist theories and treatments gave the latter an important role in maintaining psychiatry's exclusive hold over its territory: the 'normalizing' approach, by contrast, invites all and sundry to share in the task of understanding and reconciliation. As a professional ideology, then, it is a non-starter.

Yet – as Freud and Marx both held – it is possible to pay altogether too much regard to people's self-understanding; what if they are mistaken? The attempt to rely on common-sense interpretations starts to look inadvisable when we question the authority of common sense itself. We would like to be able to emulate the positivist's steely, sceptical gaze – even if we do not want to stray so far from conventional wisdom as to abandon, like him, the concept of interpretation itself. I shall suggest below that the shortcomings of the 'normalizing' approach to mental illness stem from the same fault as the shortcomings of common-sense interpretation applied to everyday life itself: namely, the inability to comprehend *compulsive* action, or *alienated* states of being.

The basic problem for any normalizing account of mental illness is a very obvious one: if the behaviour is really intelligible in common-sense terms, why was it regarded as a psychiatric problem in the first place? There are, in fact, several good answers to this question. In the first place, the decision may not have been made by an open-minded, representative sample of lay people; those responsible for it may simply have wished to invalidate the behaviour in question ('Darling, I really think you're ill!'), or they may not have had access to all the relevant information. The *context* may have been overlooked, both because traditional psychiatry lacks any way of doing justice to it, and because the people who comprise it may not wish to be implicated. The *purposes* may have been ignored because of their very nature, especially if they involve an element of protest; and the *codes* may be overlooked because of one group's ignorance and contempt towards another.

All this might explain why *some* instances of perfectly coherent behaviour get treated as symptoms of an illness; but to explain *all* psychiatric diagnoses in such terms seems a tall story. I think it has to be admitted that whatever sense is lent by a consideration of contexts, purposes and codes, there remains a residue in most 'mental illnesses' which is refractory to all ordinary procedures of understanding and empathy. After all, the 'so what' problem also applies to normalizing accounts, since by no means all who are placed in the situations we have described become 'mentally ill'; rather than leave the residue to be explained by vague and immutable 'constitutional factors', it would be preferable to see whether the concept of interpretation itself could be modified to give it greater explanatory power.

The normalizing approach exaggerates the extent to which rational free-will operates in psychiatric conditions; they are not just, as Szasz would have it, 'problems of living', but a breakdown of the problem-solving ability itself – one loses one's grip on oneself and one's grasp of what is going on.[43] Perhaps the reason why anti-psychiatrists strained so hard to deny this was that they shared with positivist psychiatry – in which tradition many of them had grown up – the belief that in such conditions, the interpretative approach breaks down altogether, and one is forced back to the 'faulty-machine' model.

But this simple opposition of free-will and determinism will not do. To avoid it, we must transcend both common sense and positivism; and this is precisely the goal of those approaches I have labelled 'depth hermeneutics', the chief of which is psychoanalysis. What is required is a way of accounting for experience and behaviour in terms of meanings, but not necessarily ones which are consciously appreciated either by the agent or his fellows; and this requires a radical revision both of our conception of the person, and of the methods of the human sciences. What has to be replaced is not only the positivist myth of man as machine, but also what Marcuse[44] calls 'the myth of autonomous man', which interpretative theorists are equally prone to. In place of the unity of the self which is assumed both by phenomenology and common sense, we must substitute Freud's conception of man as fragmented, self-contradictory, and alienated from his own experience. Only when this is done can the true meaningfulness of 'mad' behaviour become apparent – and, at the same time, the true madness of behaviour which common sense takes to be 'sane'.

Psychoanalytic approaches

In many ways the psychoanalytic approach to mental illness seems thoroughly positivistic and out of place in this chapter. Freud's basic model of the mind owed a lot to hydraulics; neurotic symptoms represented 'the return of the repressed' – that is, emotional energy which had to go somewhere after being 'blocked' by various obstacles. Superficially, too, psychoanalysis seems to generate aetiological hypotheses which relate childhood events to adult disorders in a thoroughly deterministic way. This positivistic image is entirely consistent with Freud's declared aim, which was to extend the domination of science into the last territory remaining unconquered – the human mind.

In the course of this project, however, Freud was driven ineluctably far beyond the limits of scientific orthodoxy. He himself was aware of his debt to the classical and European literary heritage, and voiced increasing uncertainty about whether his work should be classified as 'arts' or 'science'; this duality is also reflected among his followers. In America, where psychoanalysis was absorbed into the medical profession, a strictly positivistic reading was cultivated; analysts thus gained élite status and earning power, at the price of renouncing any claim to be more than emotional technologists (see Turkle and Kovel, Chapters 5 and 2). While the same marriage was attempted in Europe, it was never really consummated; it was the positivists who objected first to their new bedfellows, and only after being cold-shouldered by the medical and academic establishment did psychoanalysis seriously start to question its allegiances. Eysenck[45] was loud among those who objected to the alliance: psychoanalysis, he roundly declared, was nothing more than a revamped version of nineteenth-century *verstehende* psychology, and therefore could claim nothing in common with 'real' science. Subsequently, the English analyst Charles Rycroft[46] voiced agreement from the other side, claiming that the concern of psychoanalysis was with discovering 'meanings' and not 'causes'; since, therefore, psychoanalysis was not trying to be a science, charges that it was unscientific would (according to Rycroft) bounce off harmlessly. (We may note, for later reference, that both authors unhesitatingly accepted the equation of 'science' with 'positivism'). In

Europe, where philosophers, artists and phenomenologists had given quarter to psychoanalysis, an interpretative reading of Freud had long had currency; since the 1930s, Lacan[47] had sought to wrest psychoanalysis away from positivism, a cause which Merleau-Ponty,[48] Lorenzer[49] and Ricoeur[50] also espoused. In the U.S.A., only dissident analysts such as Szasz[51] and Shafer[52] supported such a reading. What are the grounds for calling psychoanalysis an 'interpretative' discipline? Chiefly, perhaps, because 'interpretations' are what the patient pays to get: the analyst decodes the 'latent meaning' of dreams, verbal slips, and symptoms. For Lacan, Lorenzer and Rycroft, the paradigm of interpretation was the reading of a text, and thus involved structural linguistics, semantics, rhetoric and poetics. Lacan's famous dictum 'The unconscious is structured like a language' is perhaps the best-known expression of his view: in this statement we can discern the influence of French structuralist anthropology (Lévi-Strauss, Mauss), which saw society itself as a kind of 'text' to be decoded.

What, however, is the force of the phrase '*like* a language'? In Lacan (as in structuralism generally), the analogy of language becomes a Procrustean bed, on which it is impossible to comfortably accommodate the full range of human action. The communication of a message is only one of the motives which can underlie an action; and while other motives may, like verbal meanings, exist only by virtue of a socially-maintained 'vocabulary', this does not justify cutting down the traditional concept of interpretation to a semantic sense alone. In fact, I propose to illustrate that psychoanalysis actually invokes all three of the factors which we saw utilized by the 'normalizing' approach: contexts, motives, and codes.

Like the layman, Freud first seeks to make actions intelligible in terms of their *context*; but what is distinctive about psychoanalysis is that it considers not the situation as it 'really' is, but as it is construed by the agent. It thus supplies the missing link in the theories we examined earlier, which resemble positivist accounts in that they tend to define the social context 'from outside'. Moreover, Freud is not simply invoking the situation which the agent consciously believes himself to be in, but perceptions which are for the most part unconscious. Thus psychoanalysis interprets *what situations mean to the patient*, and this is the key to its interpretation of the patient's behaviour; in this respect it resembles phenomenology, but with the crucial difference that the agent is not regarded as necessarily in touch with his own perceptions and intentions.

The notion of 'unconscious experience' (or phantasy, as the Kleinians came to refer to it) is at first sight a paradoxical one – it was thrown aside, for example, by Laing; [53] but I believe that resolving the paradox is merely a problem of distinguishing *levels* of awareness (cf. Russell's concept of 'logical types'). 'Phantasy', for a start, refers not to a sort of sideshow accompanying perceptions (though such sideshows can occur, and are very instructive to observe), but to their *structure* – the schemas or scenarios to which reality is unwittingly assimilated. Therefore, to call a phantasy 'unconscious' is merely to say that a person is unaware of the way he is construing situations, and moreover that it is so important to him emotionally to *maintain* this way of construing them that he will actively resist becoming aware of it.

A good illustration of this is 'transference' – the patient's tendency to treat the analyst as a figure from the past; the easiest way to describe that phenomenon is to say that the patient is 'unconsciously experiencing' the analytic session as (for example) a feeding relationship between mother and baby. As such identifications are made in terms of past situations – however misperceived or modified – the present is always an echo of the past; thus, for Freud, the context of behaviour is never simply the present situation, but a continuum of experience stretching back to the beginning of life.

This approach obviously has great potential for making sense of apparently inappropriate behaviour, and it provides one of the chief tactics used by psychoanalysis to 'de-reify' so-called symptoms. A man who savagely murders prostitutes may be acting quite intelligibly, in so far as he may see in the prostitutes the mother who 'betrayed' him in her sexual passion for his father; that he should see them thus is *itself* quite unintelligible without recourse to further explanation, but to see such beliefs as a sign of abnormality is to overlook the fact that the same misrecognition provides the emotional bedrock of most marriages.

Psychoanalysis also interprets behaviour by reference to its unconscious *motives* – indeed, this is regarded by most as its chief activity. I have placed 'redefinition of contexts' first, however, since this aspect of psychoanalysis is often overlooked – but the unconscious is not simply made up of motives. In fact, to redefine the beliefs informing an action is already to redefine its motive, so that one cannot properly distinguish the theory of unconscious phantasy from the theory of unconscious motivation.

Besides the notorious concept of infantile sexuality, a more fundamental motive which does not enter into the everyday vocabulary is what Freud called the 'pleasure principle', which gives rise to the phenomenon of *defences*: a person may construct an apparently pointless way of life, with the hidden aim of avoiding certain conflicts, or keeping them out of consciousness – because the 'pleasure principle' regards out of sight as out of mind, and out of mind as out of existence. One may, for example, divide the world into good and bad 'part-objects', all for the sake of avoiding the conflict of 'good' and 'bad' feelings about the same person; or one may bind oneself to another who expresses one's own unwanted feelings (the defence of 'projection'). All such defences represent an attempt to restructure the world in a more comfortable pattern – or as Freud termed it 'hallucinatory wish-fulfilment'. It is this motive which probably accounts for the phenomenon of unconscious phantasy discussed above.

The extent to which psychoanalysis invokes an unfamiliar *code* of meanings is rather more controversial. On the face of it, translation is the most obvious form of interpretation; the analogy was frequently used by Freud himself. Szasz and Lorenzer both spoke of the 'protolanguage' of symptoms, while according to Lacan,[54] the unconscious employs the literary devices of metaphor, metonymy, etc. However, as Coulter[55] and Ricoeur[56] have argued convincingly from different standpoints, it is dangerous to take this analogy with language too literally, for philosophical problems arise about the notion of 'unconscious language' which are even more awkward than those surrounding the concepts of unconscious experience and motivation. It will not do to represent Freud as simply offering a 'dictionary' of symbolic meanings; in psychoanalysis, the meaning of any symbol depends crucially on the context of its occurrence – so we are certainly not dealing with a *shared* language. In any case, a language is more than a set of symbols – it is also a way of using them; and nobody has succeeded in defining a distinctive *syntax* of the unconscious, or in explaining how such a structure could be acquired. (It could certainly not be learned, like ordinary language, by experience; how could one be 'corrected' in a task one is not even aware of performing?) Although useful as a metaphor, then, the idea of 'the language of the unconscious' is far more problematic than its devotees seem to appreciate.

The above account of psychoanalytic interpretation is, of course, incomplete and grossly oversimplified; nevertheless, it serves to indicate the kinds of praxis which analysts seek to understand, and the means they use for doing so. Actions involving *unconscious* experience or motivation cannot be encompassed either by common-sense understanding, or by mechanistic explanation; they are not under the control of the agent, but they are nevertheless meaningful. As long as the agent remains unaware of their meaning, they remain *compulsive* actions – that is, the agent does not know what he is doing, but he cannot be satisfied until he has done it. The psychoanalytic concept of 'compulsion' provides a way in which the term 'illness' may still be used meaningfully even when no organic pathology exists. Since psychoanalysis is thus concerned to enlarge the agent's sphere of freedom, Habermas characterized its interest as 'emancipatory', and took it as the model of critical social theory – theory which does not simply reproduce society's illusions about itself.

On the face of it, then, psychoanalysis seems to remedy all the defects of the 'normalizing' approach to mental illness; it is capable of interpreting the 'residue' which common sense finds unintelligible, by the apparently simple device of redefining the meaning of *situation* and *action* in subjective terms which bring the two back into coherent relationship with each other. There are two snags, however, which prevent us from rushing into the proffered embrace of psychoanalysis. One is the methodological problem, that this newly flexible concept of interpretation seems capable of encompassing everything, and therefore of explaining nothing; the other is frankly a political one, that in suggesting that mental illness is a matter of the ways in which people construe their situations, psychoanalysis tends to neglect the need to change those situations themselves. I will discuss these two problems in turn.

Methodological problems. The main objections raised by positivists against psychoanalysis have been in terms of its excessive flexibility – that it is capable of explaining everything that might happen, and is therefore unfalsifiable and unscientific (see, e.g., Popper,[57] Eysenck,[58] Borger and Cioffi[59]). The instances of 'unfalsifiability' put forward do not, however, reflect a very intelligent reading of psychoanalysis; for example, Freud's hypothesis that either a harsh or a lax upbringing would produce a strong super-ego is not 'unfalsifiable', because it excludes upbringings which are neither harsh nor lax. Specific hypotheses in psychoanalysis *are* falsifiable; and while it may be true to say that there is no crucial observation in face of which a psycho-analyst would be obliged to abandon his *general approach*, this can also be said of any other scientific system (Cosin, Freeman and Freeman[60]).

The complaint that psychoanalysis lacks explicit rules governing the *naming* of phenomena ('correspondence rules') is, however, a valid one, and this vagueness can in principle be exploited to protect the theory from falsification. In Section I, I argued for the view that correspondence rules in *any* human science are inevitably too complex to be made explicit (the 'etcetera' problem); though this implied that descriptions must always involve an element of subjective judgement, it nevertheless assumed that the judgements were constrained by *tacit* rules – those of 'common sense'.

Psychoanalysis, however, is on dangerous ground here: it cannot afford to lean too heavily on common sense, because that is precisely what it is busy undermining. The interpretations which psychoanalysts make are often *not* ones which come naturally to the layman – if they were, one would not have to pay so high a price for them; indeed, the layman is often baffled and repelled by them.

What, then, *can* psychoanalysis lean on? The predicament is not unique, nor is it anything to be ashamed of; it is shared by any theory which seeks to uncover systematic distortions in human awareness (e.g. Marxist theories of 'false consciousness'). The only solution lies in the concept of 'immanent critique': emancipatory theories (in Habermas' sense) can only seek to undermine one part of received wisdom by appeal to another – they must always be *grounded* in com-mon sense. This is only possible if common sense contains *contradic-tions* – so that the exposure of contradictions in the realm of the 'obvious' must be the essence of any 'depth hermeneutics'.

This, in fact, is an apt description of Freud's whole project. Unlike both the positivist and the mystic – who claim privileged access to a transcendent plane of 'reality', from which common sense appears as an out-and-out delusion – the psychoanalyst starts from the same criteria for interpretation as anybody else; as Shafer[61] convincingly illustrates, psychoanalytic understanding fades off imperceptibly into the everyday variety. Thus, Freud can only speak about illusion and compulsion by taking for granted the existence of true perception and free-will; he may draw the dividing-line between the former and the latter in a different place from the rest of us, but he cannot – and does not seek to – deny that the dividing-line exists at all. All this suggests, then, that the grounds on which a psychoanalytic interpretation is based must in the last resort be of a basically familiar sort, otherwise they are not grounds at all.

To sum up so far: the view that psychoanalysis is 'interpretative' does not (as Eysenck thought) remove it from the realm of science – for all human sciences must employ interpretation; nor does it (as Rycroft thought) provide a secure alternative, for psychoanalysts cannot, like theatre critics, appeal *tout court* to the obvious. I also wish to argue that to present psychoanalysis as *purely* interpretative is to miss the point of the whole exercise. As well as imputing meanings to behaviour, Freud wishes to provide a *causal* theory of how these meanings come into existence; moreover, this causal theory is essential to the credibility of the whole system, since I do not believe that without it there can be adequate grounds for making the less obvious sorts of psychoanalytic interpretation.

In a purely interpretative theory, motives and meanings are irreducible: once an action has been made conventionally intelligible, we do not seek to go beyond the account given to ask – why *this* motive? why *this* meaning? Freud, however, does precisely that, because he is concerned with people both as subjects and as objects – both acting, and being acted upon. Biology as well as history determines the particular kind of subjects which we can be: thus, in psychoanalysis the subject is 'decentered',[62] and the 'primacy of the *cogito*'[63] is abolished. This means that any attempt to eliminate causal explanations entirely from psychoanalysis turns it into something else: as Ricoeur insists,[64] 'This mixed discourse [of *force* and *meaning*] is the *raison d'être* of psychoanalysis'. Freud did not simply start off with the wrong paradigm, and correct himself as he went on – for the tension between paradigms runs through all his work; nor is Habermas[65] really justified in saying that Freud 'misunderstood himself'. Positivistic psychoanalysts may have over-estimated the causal content of psychoanalysis, but they were nevertheless right to think it was there.

This has an important bearing on the question of methodology. It is precisely his belief in certain basic *causal* mechanisms – the 'pleasure principle', for example – that gives the psychoanalyst grounds for making interpretations which common sense alone could never arrive at. But it is his interpretations that lead him to believe in the existence of these mechanisms: hence there is a subtle interlocking relationship between the two elements of psychoanalysis' 'mixed discourse', which potentially – though not inevitably – leads to circularity.

I hope I have said enough to indicate that the question we started out with – is psychoanalysis scientific? – raises vertiginous questions both about the nature of psychoanalysis, and of science – ones which serious philosophers[66] are only just beginning to confront. Moreover, the question of whether or not psychoanalysis 'works' – which is often adduced as evidence one way or the other – has to my mind very little bearing on the matter: quite apart from the problems of defining a psychoanalytic 'cure', it by no means follows that if the therapy works, the theory must be true – or vice versa (see Fisher and Greenberg[67] for an intelligent review of research on this question). All we can conclude from this section is that the methodological problems of psychoanalysis have hardly begun to be formulated, let alone solved.

Psychoanalysis and social change. Does psychoanalysis help us to understand the relationship between social conditions and mental misery, or does it merely obscure it? As we have seen, psychoanalysis helps to fill the gap in 'normalizing' approaches, by showing how an individual's *perception* of their situation may vary; but there is a very real danger that this perception will be seen as the source of the problem, rather than the situation itself. (A true story is told of a young psychoanalytic trainee who visited a woman under treatment for persecutory phantasies concerning rats: when the front door was opened, out jumped – a rat!) Psychoanalytic theory is easily used to adapt the individual to his social role, and in this guise it may become absorbed effortlessly into the repertoire of 'welfare' services. Analysis for the interesting rich; drugs or ECT for the boring remainder.

This, of course, is already to a large extent the way things are; but to accept it as an inevitable consequence of psychoanalytic theory is, I think, to read the situation back to front. Freudian theory is an account *par excellence* of the social intelligibility of mental illness; it is the brief implicit in the therapist's own role which leads to the social factors being taken as constants and the individual ones as variables – for the therapist has no mandate to change society. Unfortunately, since psychoanalytic theory has from the beginning been in the hands of therapists, its social dimension has become submerged and obscured.

The task of extracting from psychoanalysis implications for social change is one which Freud himself mostly shied away from. Some Marxists in the 1920s and 1930s were, however, anxious to do the job for him: hence arose the corpus of 'Freudo-Marxism', which includes Reich, Fenichel, Fromm, Horkheimer, Adorno and Marcuse (the last four being associated with the Frankfurt School of critical theory). Since the war, the same challenge has been taken up by many others, including Habermas, Michel Schneider, Deleuze and Guattari, and Lacan.

The early thrust of this work was to show that the institutions of capitalist society were maintained by the particular personality structure which normal child-rearing practices brought about, and thus how psychic economy and political economy supported each other. Normal personality structure was regarded as largely a system of compulsions: thus psychoanalysis was applied to the supposedly sane as well as the apparently sick, a process Freud had begun in ascribing character to neurotic mechanisms, and in his analyses of religion and mass psychology. Lacan has re-interpreted the same theme in structuralist terms by speaking of the unconscious as the vehicle of ideology – in particular, of *patriarchal* ideology ('le loi-du-père').

It is not possible to discuss this work in any detail here, but some answers may be found within it to the question posed above. On the one hand, Freudian theory has shown itself uniquely appropriate to the understanding of an irrational society, since it can account for the fact that people not only fail to recognize their own exploitation, but literally become addicted to it; a key concept here is 'internalization' of the source of exploitation. In this way psychoanalysis goes beyond the familiar limitations of the concept of 'oppression'. On the other hand, though, Freud's basic assumption was that civilization was *inherently* repressive, though I have argued – following Reich – that this is not the only way he could have interpreted his observations.[68] Furthermore, in its treatment of the family, psychoanalysis reifies the oedipal situation into a law of nature,[69] and even Lacan seems to end up by treating patriarchy similarly. Thus, although Jacoby[70] is shrill in his denunciation of 'revisionists' who tamper with Freud to make his conclusions more acceptable, it is hard to see how psychoanalytic theory can acquire a fully historical dimension without a great deal of revision. And to perform this task it is essential that the theory should cease to be the monopoly of those who maintain it for therapeutic purposes alone.

Conclusion

My purpose in this chapter has not been just to set up a marketstall of available theories of mental illness, but to bring out one central point: that no theory is value-free, each being tied to a definite commitment about social goals.

I have tried to show that psychiatry as an institution is committed to fundamentally conservative social goals, and it is this commitment rather than 'scientific' considerations that determines the choice of which theories it accepts, and which it rejects. From a different moral standpoint, I have argued that theory should be explicitly, though not exclusively, interpretative; that it must transcend common-sense understanding; and that it must incorporate social structure, not as a constant but as a variable.

The last point immediately calls in question what I have just said about psychiatry's social role. To speak of psychiatry as an 'institution' leads, in the end, to reifying it; for institutions exist not in theories but in history, and they are created and maintained by the activities of people. It is perfectly possible, therefore, for people to transform or abolish them: the example of Basaglia and his colleagues (Chapter 6) shows that mental health workers *can* – albeit not without struggle – completely redefine their allegiance and their social function, without in the process losing their specialized province. Elsewhere in this book we will return to the question of how this transformation can be accomplished.

One last point about science. In Section I, I did not bother to question whether the positivist paradigm contained, in fact, an accurate version of the methodology of the natural sciences. In a sense, however, positivism is a straw man (though still a very influential one), since what it sets out to imitate never, in fact, existed: recent philosophy of the natural sciences[71] has shown that observation *always* involves a process of interpretation, and that theories are *never* completely dictated by the 'facts'. Moreover, both cybernetics and animal biology have suggested in recent years that the special concepts supposed to be necessary for understanding human beings are relevant to the 'natural' realm as well. Thus, it is no longer obvious today, as it was to the positivists and their opponents, what exactly is implied by asserting or denying that man is a part of nature, and understandable in the same ways as nature.

All these considerations suggest that the acute division which has grown up between 'scientific' and 'humanist', or 'hard' and 'soft' approaches is not based on any *logical* distinction; *political* differences, as we have seen, exist, but once these are brought out into the open, the basis for a sharp division between paradigms for the study of man and of nature will probably disappear. At that time, hopefully, the analysis I have put forward in this chapter will become out of date: but until the political component of our disagreements is brought out into the open, we will never go beyond the phoney synthesis of psychiatric 'eclecticism'.

2 The American Mental Health Industry

Joel Kovel

Any attempt to survey the pursuit in America of what is variously called mental or emotional health runs up immediately against the sheer size of the territory and the ill-defined nature of its landscape. A dismaying prospect indeed, especially for a presentation of limited scope that must give up all claims to exhaustiveness. Surely no nation in the Western world – much less the remainder of the earth, where considerations of 'mental health' scarcely figure in social existence – can present quite the same panoply: a massive medical-psychiatric establishment; the lion's share of the world's psychoanalysts; great hosts of ancillary professionals, such as psychologists, family counselors, social workers, etc.; an interminable proliferation of alternate approaches to emotional well-being drawing on virtually every aspect of contemporary culture – in short, an entire *industry* of sorts, whose business is the production and distribution of emotional order and well-being; an industry, moreover, without substantial physical plant or readily quantifiable commodity, one subject to neither reliable objective analysis nor methodological unity, one whose separate enterprises seem to speak different languages entirely and to deal in matters that had hitherto been the province of myth, legend, superstition and the demonic. How is one to make sense of this mélange?

An approach immediately suggests itself: begin with the fact of the size, and what it calls our attention to, namely, the recent history of American society. Such a perspective is contrary to psychiatry's self-image of a medical profession whose growth is a matter of increasing mastery over a phenomenon, mental illness, which is supposed to be always present, a part of nature passively awaiting the controlling hand of science. Instead, we shall hold to the view that the disorder and the remedy are both parts of the same social process, and that they form a unity subject to the total history of the society in which they take place. The magnitude of the mental health industry, then, is not so much a sign of scientific progress as of growing contradictions in the advanced capitalist society of the United States.

(Moreover, provided one takes into account concrete distinctions beyond the scope of this essay, its principles should apply to the Western world as a whole.) This viewpoint not only serves to reveal some order in the vast and heterogeneous territories of the mental health industry; it also provides a basis for a critique of the assumptions both of the medical-psychiatric establishment and of its various competitors for the mental health market. For, as was suggested above, the one dimension repressed out of all but a handful of approaches to mental disturbance is the effect of the total society, and of the history of its modes of production and consumption, upon the emotional life of the people within it.

Although their various manifestations are endlessly intricate, the internal laws of capitalist society have imposed distinctive trends upon every sphere of social existence. This trend toward totalization is why we begin our inquiry at the level of the capitalist mode of social organization. Whatever goes on in a society will be selected and institutionally reinforced according to the degree to which it buttresses the principal mode of social production. There is no mystery in that. The only puzzle is why people are so slow to recognize this truth; or, to be exact, *how* they fail to recognize it, insofar as the reason *why* they fail to recognize it is that it is veiled from them – mystified – for a quite definite purpose. Mystification serves to buttress the prevailing mode of social organization when that mode includes domination, as capitalism most certainly does. Viewed in this light, then, the rise of a purely psychological view of human difficulties is a handy way of mystifying social reality, and it requires no feat of imagination to comprehend that capitalist society would come to reward the psychiatric profession for promoting a special kind of psychological illusion. The question still remains as to how this came to be – more precisely, in what historical sequence, in what form and with what contradictions, leading to what new developments.

The scope of the problem is too vast to admit of more than a few brush strokes by way of historical orientation. Let us pick up the thread at a time when it assumes its recognizably modern form, around the turn of the twentieth century. There is little difficulty in locating the critical period of the transition toward psychologization during the years 1905–10. There were, of course, antecedents: as a relatively unstructured society, America had long shown itself peculiarly open to experimentation with the personal sphere. The later years of the nineteenth century were rife with innovations in the psychological dimension, such as the 'mind cures' discussed by William James in his *Varieties of Religious Experience* of 1900.[1] These must be seen however as preliminary excursions into a new territory the conditions for the exploitation of which were not yet ripe. For until the twentieth century psychological enthusiasm was merely popular. There was no corresponding theory to assimilate the general interest into established forms; the medical-psychiatric profession was as a result both weakly organized and mired in a grossly organic view of mental disturbance; and, most tellingly, the state showed little interest in the problem beyond its customary concern for walling off social misfits.

All this was to crack in the latter half of the first decade of this century. Popular interest itself underwent a great surge, evinced, for example, by the doubling of magazine articles about abnormal psychology between 1905 and 1909; or by the founding of the Emmanuel movement, one of the first psychotherapeutic 'schools' in America – certainly not the last – to be developed along religious–inspirational lines.[2] More decisive however, because they revealed a turn toward institutionalization, were two other developments of the era – the founding of the Mental Hygiene Movement in 1908, and the awarding to Sigmund Freud of his honorary Doctorate of Laws by Clark University in 1909. Two years later the American Psychoanalytic Association had been founded, and within a decade psychoanalysis had proved itself, much to Freud's rue, the needed theory for bringing psychiatry out of its organic doldrums and into the twentieth century. Moreover it had fused with the ethos of mental hygiene to become the ruling ideology of medically controlled mental health – an empire that would dominate the psychological affairs of the nation until the present. In the process, psychoanalysis was to be near twisted out of shape; while the functionaries of the mental health empire, armed with their new doctrine, were to take on a quite specific twentieth-century role, compounded in equal parts of priest and technocratic expert, and dedicated to the development of a moral universe suitable for advanced industrial society.

We shall return to examine these various trends. However, no headway can be made toward their comprehension until we briefly explore the social conditions which gave them necessity. What is, after all, suitable for *this* advanced industrial society? In more useful terms, what are the peculiarities of the shift between the early and late phases of capitalism, for such is what has shaped the psychological fortunes of America – and such is what was taking a decisive turn in the very years that 'mental hygiene' made its cultural debut.

The fetish of psychology is a peculiar manifestation of late – or monopoly – capitalist society, in whose workings it plays a definite role. What makes capitalist society 'late' is the ascendency of technology – 'dead labor' – over living labor in the production process.[3] Economically this heightens the possibility of stagnation as a result of suffocation under the weight of automatically produced commodities. Capitalism adapts to the threat by a host of interrelated devices, three of which may be schematically set out here, as they shall play a continuing part in the fortunes of the mental health industry:

(1) an emphasis on the consumption of commodities

(2) increasing technical control of the human input into the production process

(3) in order to secure (1) and (2), a more or less systematic attempt to penetrate and control everyday life, including subjectivity.

It is easy to see how these efforts play into each other and serve the interests of capital in its late phase. In early capitalism, the quantity of labor time extracted in the production process was the critical variable, and the ideological apparatus of society, though crucial for the preservation of its order, was, strictly speaking, otherwise ancillary. In late capitalism, however, what is qualitative and ideological enters alongside labor time as an immediate constituent of the accumulation of capital. People have to experience the consumption of commodities as if it were a law of nature, on the one hand; while on the other, their work, increasingly remote from actual physical effort, becomes more and more a matter of supervising technical processes, watching over the sales, distribution and wasting of commodities and – of special significance – dealing with human interaction itself. Moreover, as both the imperatives of consumption and work under late capitalism go distinctly against human inclination and potentialities, the systematic invasion of private life becomes an especially compelling part of the agenda.

It should be emphasized that the inclinations and potentialities in question are not natural forms, but new possibilities opened precisely by historical development. Since the overcoming of scarcity and toil has become a real human possibility, the imperatives to labor and consume material commodities for the benefit of capital become equivalently shaking propositions. At the same time the imperatives

to labor and consume in the late capitalist mode require the development of a socially advanced population, one that is trained to a certain
degree and has enough hope to be able to want commodities but not
too much to see its way past the given order. Thus a fairly fine line is
required for the administrators of late capitalist culture. It is this
exigency that makes the invasion of private life a systematic necessity
for late capitalism. Finally, it should be emphasized that the capitalist
order has a twofold interest in technically controlling consumption,
work and daily life: first as an economic imperative to permit the
continued accumulation of capital; and second, equally important, as
a way of vitiating the capacity for organized resistance.

Concretely put, private life takes place mainly within the family,
which has consequently become a heated battleground in recent
times. This is partly a matter of the development of a child-centered
society – for childhood is the arena of desire and educability, hence a
main location for socialization in advanced capitalism. Partly, too, the
family has become so crucial an institution because of the growing
impersonality of the public sphere of work and the life of the community. As the increasing penetration by capital shrivels the public
ground upon which people can have any control over their lives,
their unmet emotional needs – which are, to be sure, cultivated
mightily by the same order which frustrates them – shift to the setting
of the family. Meanwhile, however, the family itself becomes an increasingly frail platform for social life, what with the steady loss of
parental authority (as a result, again, of the control of everyday life
exerted by capital), the exigencies of increased social mobility demanded by contemporary work, and so forth. As a result of having
to meet increased human needs with diminishing resources and
autonomy, the contemporary family has fallen into a morass of permanent crisis, an obvious indication of which is the endless stream of
neurotically crippled individuals it turns over to the mental health
industry.

Before we turn to the particular development of that industry, it
would be well to reflect a little more closely the notion of the control
of everyday life by capital, since it is the central concept of our
analysis. Until this point capital has been used in a very abstract sense
in our discussion. More concretely, we are talking about social forces
that represent the interests of capital, all of which can be summed up
under the rubric of the capitalist *state*. By the state, then, we mean the
apparatus for the administration of social life so as to allow for the

accumulation of capital and the legitimation of the social order upon which that accumulation depends. Obviously the state is a highly complex entity which may express many countervailing trends, not all of which are immediately tied to the interests of capital.[4] Certainly it goes far beyond the boundaries of government as such. In this respect we would assign some state function to those elements of society which handle key ideological functions relevant to the maintenance of capitalist relations. One would include here the managerial class of experts, along with enterprises such as advertising and the mass media, all of which have grown mightily in the contemporary era, *pari passu* with the state in general. It is through means such as this that capitalist society introduces its control of everyday life. Whether through the omnipresence of television (which has recently been defined as a necessity of life by the New York State Welfare Commission) or the experience of the supermarket, the goal is the same: destroy the chance for people to generate their own culture by systematically expunging personal control over production and consumption, and eliminating, by a capacity to seemingly absorb all opposition, any sense that people can transcend the given society.[5] Or, rather, *attempting* to eliminate opposition, since the capacity to resist remains, indeed is assured by the principal contradictions inherent to capitalist society. As the struggle for the control of everyday life develops, some of these forms of resistance may take on new aspects, including that of a subjective appearance in the guise of 'mental illness'. But of this, more later.

We may now turn to the particular group of experts who manage the mental health industry, and consider the transition of 1907–8 in the light of the foregoing analysis. Baran and Sweezy document in *Monopoly Capital*[6] that since 1907 the tendency toward stagnation inherent in the American economy has become chronic. The reasons for this are of no present concern to us; nor, in general, is the functioning of the economy since 1907, which, aided by imperialism, wars, the automobile, Keynesianism, and so forth, has more than held its own until quite recently. What is of interest is the indication that the structural tendencies that foster the development of late capitalist social relations became pronounced in the first decade of this century, and have not relinquished their hold since. In other words, any social development that would stimulate consumerism, bring work under technical control and further the penetration of daily life, would become favored by the centers of capitalist power; while any development that would enhance people's ability to take command of their social existence would become correspondingly discouraged.

Now this is not an easy program for the capitalist state. To simply crush people's ability to take command of their lives is not in itself beyond the state's capacity. If carried out overtly, however, it would result in a fascism that would undermine the state's needs to legitimate itself and, more fundamentally, be incompatible with the late capitalist accumulation process itself. Although by no means an unthinkable alternative, an authoritarian course of state action would render people incapable of either consuming or working according to advanced capitalist standards. What is suitable for a banana republic does not wear quite so well at the metropolitan center of world capitalism. But on the other hand, the simple fostering of advanced capitalist relations entails cultivation of both reason and desire – the very two elements that, in the right combination, could react to create the conditions for the overcoming of capitalism itself, with its systematic unreason and stunting of human possibilities.

As a result of these contradictions, a special kind of mystification is required of a social development if it is to pass muster in the ranks of late capitalist culture. Unreason must be dressed up as reason, and human stunting as the outcome of desire. The product of this masquerade is more than a falsified consciousness – which only connotes the promotion of illusions. No, more is involved: a very alteration of the structures of experience. The false consciousness engendered in late capitalism, then, is not merely imposed from without, by propaganda and so forth. More basically, it is secured from within, through the institution of perverted forms of rationality and desire. Because these forms have to pretend to be what they are not, the basic structures of experience, imposed at all levels of social existence, become so self-deceptive that the boundary betwen normality and what had been called 'madness'[7] ceases to exist in any recognizable shape. Since madness – whether in the form of psychosis, where the sense of reality is lost, or of neurosis, where it is retained – involves pain, disability and the threat of rebellion – it becomes a task of special significance for late capitalism to secure the boundary between madness and normality. To this frontier the minions of the mental health industry have been dispatched in ever-growing numbers. And the first expedition that was recognizably of this type was the Mental Hygiene Movement, founded in 1908, in the first flush of the capitalist state's prodigious expansion: the age of 'reform'. We may therefore single this development out from amongst the welter of developments occurring at the beginning of the century as paradigmatic of the rise of the mental health industry.

As is typically the case in our history, a manifestly benevolent and reformist tendency is seized upon for the rationalization – and hence advancement – of capitalist relations. The Mental Hygiene Movement was originally an effort to ameliorate the hideous lot of numberless people incarcerated in 'insane asylums' throughout the United States.[8] The work mainly of an ex-patient of the upper class, Clifford Beers, its first impulse was to help victims of an oppression positively medieval in its severity and neglect of human sensibility.[9] Significantly enough, a similar movement had taken root briefly in the 1880s, only to succumb to the organized hostility of organized psychiatry. Beers' venture, sparked by the phenomenal success of his autobiography, *A Mind That Found Itself*, came however at a great crest of the reformist impulse in America. It soon found the support of the most liberal and distinguished psychological minds of the day, including William James and Adolf Meyer. Even with such backing, however, the Mental Hygiene Movement languished for the first four years of its existence as it awaited connection with the main arteries of state power.[10] Then, in 1912, Dr Thomas Salmon, of the U.S. Public Health Service became associated with the organization.[11] By the time World War I came around, the connection between the state and mental health was assured. The exigencies of modern mass warfare then sufficed to make the federal government suddenly and irrevocably interested in the psychological condition of those who were doing its duty. A division of neurology and psychiatry was organized within the Surgeon General's office, with Salmon taking the role of senior consultant in neuropsychiatry to the American Expeditionary Forces. When the Rockefeller Foundation began chipping in to finance surveys by Beers' National Committee for Mental Hygiene, the circuit was closed: mental health had become a formal object for the capitalist state, and the industry designed to produce and deliver it was launched.

It is not our purpose here to explore in detail the history of the connection between the various agents of the state as they have related to mental health. Within the scope of this essay it must suffice instead to indicate the main outlines of the process, introducing only such detail as will highlight its underlying structure. For this purpose it is essential to consider the matter not only from the outward connections established between various institutions, but, equally significantly, as a function of the kind of inner discourse which serves these connections. In this respect, then, it may be said that the most signal contribution of Clifford Beers – and of Adolf Meyer, who actually suggested the term – was institutionalizing the notion of *Mental Hygiene* itself. For in so doing they provided a kind of symbolic raw material upon which the new industry could go to work.

The idea of mental hygiene had existed through most of the previous century without, however, attaching itself to more than a sporadic series of self-help manuals.[12] In other words, it had not established a substantial connection to the material conditions of social life. When conditions became ready for it to do so early in the present century, the notions of mental hygiene and health soon revealed themselves to contain a remarkable lode of symbolic possibilities for late capitalism.

The potential lay in the terms, 'hygiene' and 'health'. As substantives, they raised the level of 'mental' from that of an aspect to that of an existent thing. For an entity to have health, or be capable of hygiene, it must exist on its own in the world; it cannot merely be a quality of something else. Thus if 'mental hygiene' exists, then 'mentality' exists on its own, too; and psychology can be instituted as a distinct field of discourse, with its domain separated from the historical milieu and context in which mind develops. This kind of objectification is of course not new. Foucault, for example, documents it brilliantly throughout the eighteenth century; and it may be regarded as a facet of the development of the scientific attitude in the West. But to simply say that some development has antecedents is to miss the specifics of its historical elaboration. In any case, the special forms to which key notions such as mentality are subjected are never matters of arbitrary convenience but serve definite historical functions; and in the present case those functions can be inferred from the substantives to which mentality is yoked, namely 'hygiene' and 'health'. The two terms have overlapping implications, but with a distinction that establishes a subtle yet consequential inner relationship. They should therefore be considered separately.

Hygiene, means, to be sure, tending to promote health, but adds to it the connotation of *sanitary*. No doubt this meaning arose as a result of the great advances in public health secured through the promotion of sewer systems, plumbing, and so forth. What makes these advances significant for the mental sphere, however, is not their actuality but the objective correlate they provide for the subjective meaning of cleaning things up – repression. Hygiene in this sense links the cleansing of the mind with that of the toilets and streets: it establishes a material-symbolic link between evil, rejected wishes and thoughts on the one hand, and dirt on the other. Dirt is of course no independent substance. It is simply, as Freud held, 'matter in the wrong place'.[13] But this is, to be sure, a most profound idea, for dirt is material substance, not as the object of physics and chemistry, but as valued negatively: 'in the wrong place'. And this implies a 'right place', which, as it turns out, is the place for the accumulation of capital. If the linkage is materially established for *mental* hygiene, the same consideration for the accumulation of capital may be applied to the mental-subjective sphere as has been applied to the objective sphere. More concretely, the notion of mental hygiene, if materially grounded, provides the symbolic opportunity for linking together two functions absolutely indispensable for advanced capitalism:

(1) It allows for the objectification of emotional conditions, through the linkage with material sanitation. This not only strengthens the behavioristic tendency in psychology (which arises quasi-independently through the development of positivistic science); of more interest to us, it allows for an *exchange-value* to be placed on states of mind. In other words, condition A (which may be correlated with a mental 'disease' – see below), can be measured and determined to be so much worse than condition B; and the distinction A–B can be made equivalent to the expenditure of a quantity of time and/or money. Thus clinical-psychological work – including, to be sure, psychotherapy – can take its place in the general framework of capitalist relations; standards of accreditation and accountability can be instituted where the state (or insurance companies) provides payment; and, in short, the economic basis of the mental health industry becomes securely anchored in capitalist society.

(2) Mental hygienics provides the very means of dealing with deviant behavior that capital has been waiting for. As it moves into its late phase, capital must, for reasons outlined above, increase consumption and the technical control of social reality. Moral imperatives – and the entire religious framework which gave them vitality – have to be slackened in the interests of a new permissiveness; while social control – as necessary as before – must become correspondingly instrumental and invisible. No better way exists for capital to meet these exigencies than to institute 'health ethics' in general, and the notion

of mental hygiene in particular, as the paramount criterion of what is socially desirable or deviant. In the new order, people are no longer undesirable, bad, mad or possessed: they are *sick*, and need the ministrations of a mental hygienist, the technically skilled, impersonal practitioner of a remunerable skill. And if they get too sick, they have to be put away, for their own good, or society's.

The notion of mental hygiene, then, secures in one swoop both the commodification of mind and the technical control of deviance through its linkage of health with sanitation. Why therefore bother with a separate consideration of mental 'health'? The answer is revealed by a glance at the history of the practice of mental hygiene. For it is not sanitary engineers who have dominated the institutions of the mental health industry, but physicians. It is to the medical profession that the clean-up job has been entrusted; and it is into the medical categories of health and disease that the history of mental hygiene has been subsumed.

There is clearly no mystery in this, since physicians had been, along with the clergy, entrusted with forbidden personal matters for centuries; while unlike the clergy, they had also been securing a kind of technical mastery over the realm of health. The reform era, during which the mental hygiene movement was born, witnessed also the inception of the American medical profession in its modern form. Again, control of an abuse led the way to the consolidation of state power. In this instance the abuse was the proliferation of medical training institutions, many of which did not come up to reasonably scientific standards. The reform was the Flexner report of 1910 (underwritten by the Carnegie Foundation) which established the basis for stringent control over medical education and licensure, and led to the creation of the technocratic medical élite that has dominated American health affairs since. The older system, for all its flaws, permitted wide access to medical training from a number of social classes, not to mention women and minority groups. Suddenly, in the second decade of the twentieth century, medicine had been transformed into an upper-middle-class white male preserve, its economic power secured by control of the supply of doctors, on the one hand, and of the ideology which determined the demand for medical services, on the other.

The details of the development of the American medical profession need not concern us here. What counts is its hegemony – greater, perhaps, than for any other nation, owing to the disproportionate role technocracy has played in American life, and the fervid belief Americans have had in environmental meliorism. Surely, this belief has run, the physician, with his mysterious and esoteric mastery of the body, would be able to bring about the conquest of illness, and with it, eternal life and happiness. Such a function can – and was – readily transferred to the care of the mind through the symbolic construction of mental hygiene and health. Thus was psychiatry established as the pre-eminent interest in the mental health industry, a dominance it holds onto tenaciously still, despite all the intricate developments and challenges of recent decades.

Before describing some of these developments, it might be worthwhile to explore a bit further into the peculiarities of medical hegemony over mental health care, including some of the reasons why it has proven so successful in squelching alternate perspectives despite the manifest inability of American psychiatry to do more than tinker with the extreme edges of the problem it addresses. We are not disputing here that this tinkering has been of some real value. There is no question, for example, that the bulk of suffering and disability imposed by severe psychosis has been lessened through the widespread use of tranquillizing and antidepressant drugs (in contrast to neurosis, where drugs have by and large only made matters worse), or that some definite advances have been made in hospital care as a result of the continued working of the reformist impulse. As with the rest of the culture of capitalism, one misses the point entirely by denying to psychiatry any and all virtue or progress. The question is rather: why the *mystique*? – especially when the progress achieved has been so meagre relative to the effort expended and human possibilities for something better; and moreover has been accompanied by so much inattention to social needs, not to mention waste, false privilege, mediocrity and dehumanization. Why, in short, have people been willing to settle for so little?

If there is an answer to the question, it must be composed of several intertwined strands. At the risk of being schematic we may isolate a few.

(1) *The suppression of an alternate vision of society.* It is anything but accidental that the period during which the mental health industry became medically instituted coincided with the high-water mark of American socialism – and, needless to add, with the first triumphs of international socialism. And if there is one factor which dialectically accounts for the success of American psychiatry it is the failure of

American socialism. The political weakness of the American working-class movement and its susceptibility to being bought off and distracted are not our province here.[14] But psychiatry should be singled out as both an instrument and a beneficiary of this distraction: an instrument, both in its general function as well as its more particular employment in industry as a means of cooling off workers;[15] and a beneficiary, insofar as the failure of American socialism (coupled with the demise of religions) left the desire for transcendence which it had represented no place to go other than the personal sphere. This territory was being eagerly cultivated during the 1910s and 1920s by advertising and media – as it has been even more assiduously cultivated in recent decades – and psychiatry, purveyed as a bonanza of personal meliorism, was and remains in a highly favored position for exploitation.

(2) *The promotion of a professional establishment.* The 'professionalism' upon which so much of the prestige of medicine and psychiatry rests depends upon massive institutional arrangements. These arrangements determine the power of a profession, and its social influence, in a way that is only incidentally related to the value of its services. The institutional base of a profession is responsive primarily to its inner politics and ultimately to the social power residing in the capitalist state. Those served by the profession are only secondarily involved – and in the case of psychiatry, which deals in what is socially objectionable, only a minimal input from consumers takes place. Therefore the immediate reason for the hegemony of medical psychiatry is readily found in the hermetic power of its institutions. These are complex and interlocking. They consist of a large network of training centers, primarily at medical schools or various state-funded treatment centers; the treatment settings themselves, both private and state-run hospitals; professional societies, the most important being the American Psychiatric Association, which looks out for the welfare of psychiatry; powerful industrial interests, especially the pharmaceutical business, directly involved in the purveyal of mental health and closely identified with the medical profession; foundations and other quasi-public agencies; and – last but certainly not least – the state regulatory agencies themselves: the various state departments of mental hygiene, the federal National Institute of Mental Health, and the powers behind them.

This is a fairly seamless empire, almost exclusively responsive to its own needs as an institutional network, no matter how much individuals working within it may separate themselves from its imperatives. The empire controls training, academic promotion, licensure, accreditation, the dispersal of research grants, funding for services and professional journals. Needless to add, all of these activities are defined in a way that reinforces medical hegemony. The only points in the system in which a non-medical presence can be introduced are at the level of government agencies. These have been until the present quite thoroughly controlled by medical interests, however.

The perpetuation of medical hegemony is almost incidental to the sheer mass of this institutional empire and its capacity to define the reality of mental health care in America. Unless one believes that bureaucratization of this scope is a liberating influence, the spectre it raises is a somber one indeed. Although many medical or non-medical people who work within American psychiatry are motivated by humane therapeutic goals and/or a spirit of scientific inquiry, the degree to which they can realize these aims is limited at every point by the mental health bureaucracy. For the mental health industry as a whole cannot and will not go beyond the exigencies of advanced capitalist relations. Furthermore, political awareness within it is minimal. Reform is correspondingly superficial, and resistance sporadic and unorganized. Therefore all who work for it experience constraints on whatever they would like to do in a humane, genuinely scientific and unalienated way, constraints considerable enough to render any breakthrough an individual, almost an accidental, phenomenon.

We should remind ourselves here that the historical detail has been left out of this section. The important fact to bear in mind is that, despite all particular developments, one overarching trend is unmistakable: in the little more than a half-century of its existence, the medical arm of the mental health industry has not simply grown absolutely in size but, more significantly, has continually become more dependent upon and intertwined with the state. This should come as no surprise to any observer of modern society, but as it runs against the grain of medicine's self-image as a professional guild of small independent businessmen, it deserves emphasis, especially as the relationship portends so much for the future. We may now consider the third strand of the hegemony of medical psychiatry.

(3) *The medical model of mental illness.* The most conspicuous point at which the mental health establishment sets its constraints upon the development of a genuinely scientific and liberating approach to emotional disorder is the ideology of the medical model.

The medical model of mental illness completes the reification inherent in the notion of mental hygiene by bringing mind (or behavior, or personality), viewed now as a substance, under the sway of medical technics. This has an obvious cultural power, since it combines in one conception the mystique of the machine and the managerial ethos. In its system the doctor-expert is the manager of the soul, regarded now as a mechanism like any other, capable of tuning up or overhauling. Care is defined in a top-down direction, the patient, quiescent as any machine, accepting the ministrations of the expert technician. The notion also has a political power, since what is repressed out of the medical model of mental illness is that dimension which considers the person an active social agent, defined by what class, community, and history have meant for him. What is left after the excision of this dimension is the idea of individual as monad, a container holding the mechanisms of personality within itself and surrounded by an environment consisting of other monads. Accordingly, disease is something going on within a person; it is to be looked for in the malfunctioning of the 'parts' of his personality and not in the entire relationship between the self and the world; and it is to be remedied by individual or particularistic action. Lacking a sense of history, the medical model inevitably slides into biological types of explanation. Society becomes just another part of the environment impinging upon the individual: a 'factor'. Its influence is considered to be mainly quantitative, along the model of physical 'stress', i.e. too much noise, effort, fumes or too little reinforcement, support or whatnot. How the social world functions as a totality, how it draws the individual into it, what the world *means* to a person, and how people relate inter-subjectively to each other – all this becomes foreign to the medical model.

It should not be thought that social problems are beyond the scope of the medical model. Quite the contrary: the model exists to gobble them up and medicalize them. What is beyond the model is the connection with the reality of capitalist society. More precisely, one of its functions is to repress out this connection so that problems of social origin appear assimilable to the prevailing technocracy. Indeed the medical model in psychiatry must, by its own dynamic, steadily encroach on more social territory.[16]

No pursuit is dearer to medical psychiatry – nor fills its time more busily – than the search for diagnostic accuracy, indeed, perfection. Diagnosis is the Holy Grail of official psychiatry and the key to its legitimation. The medical model demands classification of its monads along the order of somatic medical disease or any other set of physical objects. If this cannot be accomplished, then the whole model breaks down, since the presence of an additional dimension which tends to dissolve the mechanistic conception of personality will have been disclosed. On the other hand, if a system of diagnosis can be sustained, so much the better for the authority of medical psychiatry, which can continue to exert ideological control over social deviance by telling people that they have a case of this and not that, and to impose from on high an appropriate treatment plan. If it should turn out in reality, furthermore, that the effort to diagnose people from a medical-psychiatric standpoint is a hopeless charade and not serious science, then one might also expect the psychiatric establishment to rush great numbers of stalwart researchers to the breach, while at the same time redoubling its efforts to promote the meaningfulness of its classificatory schemes. And the result is as expected, since as any unencumbered look at human disorder will reveal, the only thing which permits the medical-style classification of emotional disturbance is superficiality of thought and observation.[17] By the same token, any real knowledge of a person reveals him or her to be set into a system of relationships remote from the static and ahistorical schemata of official diagnosis.

But instead of following reality official psychiatry has redoubled its efforts to conjure up a new chimera. Currently the American psychiatric world is breathlessly awaiting the outcome of a veritable Manhattan Project to clear up the mystery of diagnosis once and for all: the American Psychiatric Association's DSM-III. Word is out that this new and definitive Diagnostic and Statistical Manual has made several neat carvings into the world of schizophrenia, eliminated neurosis as a category, and discovered new species of personality type for the purpose of labelling, e.g., the 'avoidant personality'. That the psychiatric establishment is not a total monolith unresponsive to consumer pressure is shown by the hotly contested abandonment of homosexuality as a disease entity. To what extent this has been a result of pressure from the gay community, to what extent a reflection of the increasing permissiveness of consumerist mass culture, is not a matter we can adequately investigate here. That the change should be hotly contested deserves some note, however; for what is at stake is more than emotional prejudice. To weaken the bonds of diagnosis means both that some portion of behavior hitherto deemed sick, and hence deviant, is now relatively more accepted; at the same time it tends to weaken the economic hold of those who have established the right to treat people so long as they can be defined to have a disease. As the mental health industry anxiously anticipates National Health Insurance – which can potentially disrupt the established order of remuneration – the battle over diagnosing can only sharpen. DSM-III must be seen then as American psychiatry's attempt to roll with the times and anticipate the challenge to its authority.

That authority may be expected to have an increasingly difficult time asserting itself in the period ahead. Not the least of psychiatry's problems is the intellectual rot induced by long years of having to defend the gap between the medical model and reality. It may even be – though this is to a certain extent speculation – that the gap is widening. It could be that the model once provided some simulation of human reality – say, in the beginning of the late capitalist period – but that it becomes increasingly irrelevant in so-called post-industrial society, so that disturbance patterns have indeed become more diffuse under the impact of today's culture. Such may or may not be the case. What is indisputable however is the banality of outlook required to seriously believe that people really conform to official psychiatry's vision of them. Authority may be retained thereby – provided the state goes along, which may of course be taken for granted under the present society. However, the costs at the level of theory and practice are great and growing; [18] and so, despite all its power, the empire of medical psychiatry rests on a crumbling base.

The medical model owes some of its longevity to a feature of emotional disorder as yet unexamined by us, namely, its horrific character. Whatever the elusive phenomenon may be in an ultimate sense, madness as lived in everyday life invariably entails unbearable pain and terror. There is probably no more cogent way of conceptualizing the different forms of emotional disturbance than as different strategies of mitigating anxiety, usually by a distortion of consciousness. It follows therefore that, whatever their socio-economic function, models of emotional disorder will tend to be selected for the way they help people repress the truth about themselves as much as for the way they help account for some portion of reality. The medical model, precisely because of its naïve positivism, is in itself an anodyne against self-realization, and so will be accepted all the more readily for the illusions it promotes.

But if this be the case, then what must be the fate of psychoanalysis, the tradition that looms largest in the development of twentieth-century American psychiatry, and which was itself founded on the assumption that the demonic terrors behind the façade of consciousness could be unmasked and subjected to rational investigation? Freud's greatness is dialectically compounded out of scientific power and the courage to face up to the unbearable. The former gave him a critical eye, and the latter, strength to probe the depths where he found – not as a matter of theory but as an actual living fact of the social process – both hatred and desire in fantastic excess beyond what the social order deemed acceptable. In order to keep its eyes open to the depths then, psychoanalysis *necessarily* has to adopt a deeply critical attitude toward society. Depth psychology cannot be itself unless it is linkable – at least in principle – to a radical political attitude. Although easily overlooked, this remained the case for Freud, who, despite his pessimism and personal conservatism, never really took the side of the established order, indeed, could write as late as 1927 that 'a civilization which leaves so large a number of its participants unsatisfied and drives them into revolt neither has nor deserves the prospect of a lasting existence'.[19]

But depth psychology can only be linkable to political attitudes of any kind. The connection is not prearranged; it develops along with the psychology and, in developing, leaves an indelible mark on psychological theory and practice. In the case of psychoanalysis, some strange things were to happen to Freud's thought as it seeped into American culture.

The story is far too complex to be treated fully here. However, a few of its features are of particular interest. One should especially note the substantial interval between Freud's visit of 1909 and the major influx of Hitler-driven European analysts which began in the 1930s. It was only after the latter immigration that psychoanalysis began taking on its Mandarin status within the mental health professional empire. And one reason for the élitism was the discovery, made by the European analysts on their arrival, that they had come upon a culture which had been digesting their doctrine for a whole generation and turning it to its own purposes.

As Hale[20] points out, the problem started with Freud at the time of his visit. Although it is well enough known, the fact that Freud's thought underwent many major developments from the beginning of his psychoanalytic career to the end is generally not sufficiently appreciated. In any event, the psychoanalysis Freud presented to America in 1909 – and seemingly embellished, for reasons of his own

– was a long way from the stoical and conservative doctrine of his latter years. It was, rather, full of therapeutic optimism and a rather unusual emphasis on environmental influence [21] – enough of an emphasis to permit the interpretation that emotional disturbance could be readily cleared up by bringing the unconscious to consciousness, whereat it could be condemned by the waking, civilized self and/or 'sublimated' into socially acceptable pursuits.

Just how much of an opportunity Freud left open for such an interpretation – shorn as it was of the notions of resistance and transference, indeed of any problematic or radical view of mind – is a somewhat moot point. What matters is that it was just such an interpretation of psychoanalysis upon which the Americans seized and avidly began to elaborate in their own fashion. In the Americanized version of psychoanalysis Freud's breathtaking insights into the psychological depths became instantaneously banalized. The unconscious became more like sludge than anything else: something that could be dredged up and dumped somewhere else. And the ego-forces that did the dredging were correspondingly aggrandized, along with the conformist tendencies of society, for it was society that ultimately commanded the authority to condemn and the paths to sublimation.

The key point is this: psychoanalysis took hold in its Americanized version because capitalist society was in the process of demanding a moral transformation of a certain kind when Freud happened to come along and was found suitable. What was great in Freud – his critical ability to see beneath, if not beyond, the established order – was necessarily jettisoned; while what was compatible with advanced capitalist relations – the release of a little desire, along with its technical control and perversion – was as necessarily reinforced. The seamless repression of the old organic model was passé in a world where the administration of everyday life was fast becoming an economic necessity for capital. What the managers of society selected instead was a doctrine that permitted the registration of psychological relations and the expression of impulse, only to trap them in a net of banality. Psychoanalysis became the sought-after coping-stone insofar as it combined a biological base with a pragmatic attention to the realities of everyday life as they were registered subjectively. And as Hale points out, it was the only systematic psychology of the time that paid real attention to the moral sphere. Finally, its subversive tendencies proved easily submersible beneath the weight of class-interest.

Within a decade of Freud's visit, then, psychoanalysis in America had become near-totally accommodated to the categories of mental hygiene. The American Psychoanalytic Association, few of whose first members were psychoanalysts in any recognizable sense, had already become what it remains to this day – a medically-dominated guild. Popular and scientific writings were meanwhile converging on the way this new form of confessional would not only stamp out madness but bring positive happiness as well – happiness defined now, as the title of one of the books of the time had it, as 'Moral Sanitation'. Sublimation in socially acceptable tasks was heavily stressed, including that most acceptable of tasks: work. And mental hygienics converged perfectly with the rise of scientific management, W. Alanson White concluding that the psychoanalyst's goal should be to assure maximum 'output'.[22]

In the following decade of the 1920s, the penetration between hygienic psychoanalysis and the corporate order became a two-way process with the discovery that the new psychology could be used as a key instrument for the shaping of desire in the age of consumerism. With Edward Bernays, Freud's nephew and the founder of modern public relations, leading the way,[23] the advertising industry began making use of the new psychology to market fetishized desires. (Their first triumph, for which the leading popularizer of Freud, A. A. Brill, played a consulting role, was to get women to smoke). Although the immediate effect on psychoanalytic thought of such shenanigans – which continued on and off thereafter – was slight, the eventual impact has been profound. For penetration of this sort locks a certain form of theory and practice into mass culture: it makes a banal, conformist psychoanalytic ideology into much more than a clinical formulation, indeed, makes it an imperative for the most 'advanced' form of capitalist relations.

One should not overdraw the picture and lose sight of its constructive as well as negative elements during this era. Certainly of the former there were – and continued to be – numerous examples. With its enthusiasm, willingness to innovate and headstart in exploring the mind, America was bound to be the site of many original contributions; for example, the work of Harry Stack Sullivan who, in these same 1920s, became perhaps the first to really grasp the idea of schizophrenia as a human experience, and developed many insights into the social origins of neurosis. But there is less need to emphasize positive individual achievements than the easily forgotten societal context in which they were carried out. For it is the social order – with its imposition of conformism and shallowness, and the loomings of bureaucratic state control, that is destined to play the decisive role in the absence of organized conscious resistance. And by the 1930s, the fetish of psychology demanded by late capitalism had firmly taken root in American soil.

Such was the domestic spectacle that greeted the European Freudians when they reached these shores. Their response, as noted above, was to mandarinize psychoanalysis, to preserve its pure gold against the dross they saw all around them. In view of the foregoing analysis, a rationale for the maintenance of a rigorous approach to psychoanalysis is not hard to find. If there is a more or less systematic, although unarticulated, cultural attempt to banalize a doctrine, then those with a feeling for its depths have a right to protect its integrity through careful control of training, methodology, and so forth. If one takes the unconscious seriously, then psychoanalysis has to be a painstaking, exacting and time-consuming therapy carried out by people who have themselves been analysed. Indeed, for all the necessary limitations, the value of psychoanalysis as a form of treatment has, if anything, grown because of the premium it places on self-reflection in a culture increasingly hostile to deep thought of any kind.

But a rationale for a course of action need not be the whole reason for it. Without gainsaying the legitimacy of the motivations *within* psychoanalytic discourse that led the Freudians into their élitist ways, it remains necessary to point out motivations kept *outside* of psychoanalytic discourse which contributed greatly to the same end. There was of course nothing mysterious about this latter level. It was – and remains – nothing other than class interest, for the pure gold of psychoanalytic treatment has only been made available to those who had coin to exchange for it, not to mention leisure and sophistication. And although psychoanalysts are in general no more than comfortable economically, and probably earn less (by virtue of being only able to treat a small number of patients) than other medical or psychiatric colleagues, the prestige that accrues as a result of their highly developed skill further establishes their class position in the upper echelons of American society.[24]

Despite their élitism, American psychoanalysts never got far out of touch with the main body of the mental health professional establishment (which indeed serves psychoanalysis, in today's leaner years, with a great proportion of its patient population). In direct opposition to Freud's wishes,[25] the profession established itself firmly in the camp of medicine. When, therefore, the mental health industry began its great boom in the post-World War II era, psychoanalysts were able to play key roles in the many burgeoning training programs that arose in this period. This worldly contact has posed a number of problems of psychoanalysis, but it has done nothing to weaken the medical tone of the profession, which leaves its mark on many levels of theory and practice. With the advent of national health insurance, the medical connection of psychoanalysis – not to mention its professional bureaucratization – is bound to become intensified.

American psychoanalysis is today an uneasy hybrid, its high degree of clinical sophistication trapped and bogged down by a theory which is heavily influenced by the medical model of mental illness. That this should occur comes as no surprise when it is realized how much history has had to be repressed out of psychoanalytic thought because of the unexamined class position of the analysts. Here again the function of an ahistorical medicalized model becomes evident. We noted above that analysts justify their élitism by looking within their theory for the 'pure gold' they feel it preserves. Meanwhile they correspondingly ignore their class interests as a motivation. It follows then that the theory is constructed to facilitate this split. Repression is carried out within the theory itself by its postulation of deep infantile fantasy as the prime mover of the self and its ignoral of the way such fantasy is shaped and realized by its intersection with the world of history. There is no better way to get a blank stare than to introduce the question of class interest to a gathering of American psychoanalysts. The reason is obvious, but ignored: to consider class interest would be to call too much into question – not just practice, but the self-image of the disinterested scientist. What is at stake is the very reality principle uncritically upheld by contemporary psychoanalysis, that of the bourgeois order. Indeed, psychoanalysts have even by and large forgotten their own history, failing to recognize that certain pillars of analytic orthodoxy, for example Otto Fenichel, were at the same time Marxists who recognized the need to bring the two points of view into apposition.[26]

While its own élitism kept psychoanalysis on a narrow if comfortable base, the enormous surge of post-war interest in questions of mental health soon caused it to be outflanked. As the New Deal completed the consolidation of monopoly power with the state, the post-war era saw a consumerism scarcely dreamt of by turn-of-the-century planners. Thus all of the influences fostering the growth of psychologism were augmented; older channels by which psychological needs had been met soon overflowed; and new ones grew to meet the demand. We shall focus on two broad areas of contemporary demand for mental health services: (1) neo-reformist social psychiatry, and (2) the new, humanistic psychotherapies.

(1) *Neo-reformist social psychiatry*. The more than a million men rejected by the armed forces in World War II for 'mental unfitness' called attention to the immense degree of crippling exacted by life in advanced industrial society. These trends, needless to add, only mounted as personal life crumbled under the assorted strains increasingly placed on it by the age of administered social existence. On top of all this, emotional disorder becomes much more glaring in the complex and fragmented world of late capitalism than it would be in earlier modes where a reasonably intact local community provides support and protection. As the state in capitalist society has destroyed local community life, so has the state picked up the need to provide human support functions. This it attempts to do in its fashion, mediating between the citizenry and power interests, and eventually settling for bureaucratic dehumanization.

In the post-war era the heightened needs for emotional care were at first met by an unresponsive medical-psychiatric élite devoted to individual private practice on the one hand and, on the other, the same massive and subhuman state hospital system which society had fitfully been trying to reform for a century. The time was therefore ripe for another effort at reform. Although the development of tranquillizing drugs in the 1950s had taken some of the pressure off the state hospital system, scarcely a dent had been made in the real problem. Indeed the spectre of emotional disability seemed to grow under the eyes of those who attempted to administer care. In part this had to do with rising expectations in the population, who were suddenly being told that the miseries they had immemorially endured could now be scientifically helped. From another angle, it is the inevitable result of the logic of the mental health model which, having to keep real social forces submerged, necessarily expands the domain of suffering it addresses, until it pretends to help not only madness but all forms of unhappiness and social discontent, from alcoholism to crime and even poverty.

In any event, the post-war era was a time of a rapid increase in attention to psychological unhappiness. Given the inelasticity of established institutions, new ones were bound to arise. In a premonitory way, the state recognized this by establishing the National Institute of Mental Health in 1949. Despite its mandate to attend to the mental health needs of the community at large, the NIMH passed the first fifteen years of its existence cosily controlled by the medical-psychiatric establishment, under whose auspices it spent the great bulk of its monies funding research and other academic pursuits.

In the 1960s, however, the wave of reform struck. Spurred in part by reformist elements within the psychiatric profession (such as the Group for Advancement of Psychiatry), in part by growing pressure for participation by citizens, and enthusiastically backed by the Kennedy administration, the age of *community* psychiatry was launched. The centerpiece of the new mode was the Community Mental Health Center (CMHC). Partially funded by federal legislation in 1963 (and also supported by states and municipalities), the number of these locally-based centers for the delivery of mental health care has grown to roughly four hundred, serving approximately one million clients in 1972.[27]

A venture of such size, involving so many conflicting interest groups, and still in the process of formation, resists ready summarization. However, a few broad conclusions can already be drawn. One is that the community mental health movement has presented a definite threat to the hegemony of the medical-psychiatric establishment; moreover, it provided the possibility, and in a few instances the realization, for politicizing of emotional care. For the first time in the history of American psychiatry, some inroads had been made from the underside – from consumers and from hitherto lowly non-medical staff.[28] And for the first time, some cracks had been made in the medical model of mental hygiene. Perhaps the most notable advance has been made by providing superior alternatives to hospitalization (which is of course inherently under medical control) through various outpatient programs to deal with crises, the chronically psychotic, and so forth.

But cracks can be healed, particularly if recuperative power still resides with the affected agent. And since the community mental health movement was never more than an attempt at liberal reform – i.e. since funding and accrediting power always remained with the NIMH and the state in general – there need never have been serious question as to which side would eventually prevail. As critics of the movement pointed out all along,[29] the grandiose social schemes of the community movement never really left the umbrella of the medical-psychiatric model in the first place. Moreover, when the community got out of hand and began demanding real power (as for example in the Bronx's Lincoln Hospital in 1969[30]), two rather predictable things occurred. First, chaos ensued, since even such stretched categories of mental health care as the community movement flaunted could not accommodate a transfer of political power; and second, the state stepped in and put a halt to the experiment – more precisely, saw to it that 'community psychiatry' would get channeled back into safe bureaucratic ways.

Indeed, although most of the CMHCs have been safe, and even tepid, organizations, the general rightward swing of public policy in the 1970s has seriously undermined the power of the movement as a whole. We are told that President Carter and his wife are strong advocates of the mental health movement. Whether this signals a change in its fortunes remains to be seen. But whatever the fate, the overall verdict has to be guarded. The harsh judgment has been made that community mental health means 'nothing for everyone'. This falls well short of the truth, for some real increase in access to needed services has occurred, and there are a number of facilities which provide superior care, but it suggests the way things have drifted: away from authentic participation and toward faceless bureaucracy. In certain New York State facilities now, for example, workers are no longer called therapists but 'case managers'. The shift in terminology is associated with the fact that for many of them work consists more of filling out forms than of contact with people. This transition, which repeats the basic movement of late capitalism – dead labor over living – is therefore anything but superficial. It reflects not so much the overcoming of the medical model as its inherent unfolding toward dehumanization. The medical-psychiatric model must deny the social activity of people by labelling their disturbance as a disease inside them that can be treated from the outside by an expert from the upper classes. Faced with a democratizing threat such as community participation, the inner structure of the model is retained by the state at the expense of its outer shell. The role of therapist retains the possibility of a real human dialogue that could indeed overcome the alienation inhering in the hygiene model. That of manager, however, restores the distance proper for late capitalist relations.

The reproach is easily levelled at the community mental health movement that it has been done in by 'politics' – by internecine squabbles, petty deals over who is going to control the grants and other funds, and so forth. The above analysis shows how superficial this criticism is (indeed it is often made in the interests of restoring professional élitism). 'Politics' in the abstract is not the issue, but the particular politics spawned by the contradictions of the capitalist state. It would be better to say that community mental health has been done in by an *insufficient* politics – a politics without vision or grasp of the true social forces at play. Read through a standard compendium of community mental health theory and practice,[31] and you will be immediately struck by the lack of serious attention to how society itself works. Given such shortsightedness, the 'community' – or, as it is officially called in a term that splendidly evokes the state's intent, the 'catchment-area' – loses all structure, becoming instead a collection of atomized individuals serviced by another collection of bureaucrats,[32] whose ranks would soon be swelled by mental health functionaries.

(2) *The new psychotherapies.* Among the more significant stimuli introduced by the post-war reform movement were demands for a more accessible and pragmatic psychotherapy than that practiced by psychoanalysts. With general systems theory for a base, one main current of this new impulse has taken the shape of family therapy, while others were realized in a great expansion of various group approaches.[33] The new modes were logically suited for community mental health practice, hence thrived with the movement and remain one of its more valuable legacies. Unhappily these therapies are suited to community mental health in its shortcomings as well as its strengths. While permitting rapid engagement with emotional reality, family therapy has tended to settle for a shallower, more immediate grasp, leaving out of account both deep unconscious individual influences and deep social ones. In this respect, systems theory, while promising a transcendence of the medical model, has only shifted its object from the molecule of the individual to the cell of the family, once more leaving the larger body of society out of focus. By training its sights on 'communications', the prevalent systems theory helps practitioners ignore the reality that forces communication of a pathological kind. The existing family – with all its repressive and conformist tendencies – inevitably becomes seen as an end in itself instead of the plaything of larger societal forces; social systems become extended families, or 'networks';[34] and an ultimately psychological causation is substituted for history.

This notion – that feeling, mind, the self, or whatever cognate can be advanced to describe purely psychological relations, is to be considered the primary factor in the human situation – has become a ruling passion of contemporary late capitalist culture. Fed by all the resources of advertising and mass media, it is part of the vision of the good life of consumption, a life built out of administered pleasure. There is nothing more natural in this scheme of things than that an improved self should be administered, too; and so, as the age of consumption waxed, the era of psychotherapy reached its zenith, promising a new wave of mind cures. The distinction between the earlier craze and the current one is as important as the continuity, however. Where the initial surge was a largely spontaneous populist movement, today's version is big business, and organized: supported by a powerful media apparatus and hooked into consumer culture.[35] The difference represents the integration of mental health as a commodity-form.

A twofold stimulus lies behind the rise: the increase in neurotic misery as a result of alienation and the collapse of the family on the one hand and, on the other, a demand for the more meaningful existence both promised and denied by late capitalism. As the community psychiatry movement responded essentially to working-class demands, the new era of psychotherapy is basically a phenomenon for those better off. With stomachs full and hearts empty, such people are now promised, in the guise of therapy, the humanity erased from social existence by history. Hence the overarching rubric of the movement – the *humanistic*, a term applicable whether the therapy in question involves talking, screaming, feeling, massaging, meditating, touching, rebirthing, or any of the possible pathways to self-realization, i.e. so long as it stays within the limits of the prevailing psychologism.

This is not the place to detail any of these modes, which are treated individually elsewhere, both as to their techniques and hidden ideology.[36] The reason is less a matter of limited space than of indicating the unity of the approaches for all their seeming diversity and rabid competition. When primal therapy proclaims itself superior to gestalt, and bioenergetics to both, we are not witnessing anything fundamentally different from the competition obtaining between, say, Ford and Chrysler. Each of these enterprises is competing for a segment of a market, and their theory and practice stray as little from capitalist ways as do those of any business.[37] As for being revolutionary, it should be recalled that auto manufacturers call their new models revolutionary, too.

To be sure, there have been genuine probes toward spontaneity in recent times, which in themselves contain a movement toward liberation. But nothing remains in itself within capitalist culture: it either gets trapped, drawn back into the prevailing mode, or it resists. Lacking resistance, any revolutionary pretense is mere public relations. There are, to be sure, instances where such resistance has occurred. As with psychoanalysis, most of the newer therapies can be – and have been – practiced with an eye toward political emancipation. The goal here is to employ the therapy to free up bound personal energies so as to permit the individual to make real demands on the world. At the same time, the therapy must be able to permit one to achieve solidarity with others in the same cause. It is a difficult business, still at the fledgling stage and, unhappily, yet a minority position. For as a rule, the new therapies have shown as little inclination to resist as the older psychoanalytic ones. As a result they thrive blithely for a while, then either get replaced by a new model or lapse into rigid formalism and/ or bureaucratization.[38] Eventually, if a new therapy really amounts to something, it will be used – as psychoanalysis was by advertising in the 1920s – to serve the state directly. Such has been the fortune, for example, of Transactional Analysis (TA),[39] the group-treatment method of which has been drawn upon by corporations, the military and even prisons, as a way of promoting greater harmony among their subjects.

Finally we may briefly consider the various radical, or antipsychiatry alternatives to the established forms of emotional treatment. Briefly, because for all the importance of the issues it raised, radical psychiatry never really took hold in America and has proven one of the most perishable of New Left movements.

The reason radical psychiatry succumbed so readily to the repressiveness of the 1970s is that it consistently failed to realize the extent of the problem it was addressing. By missing the totality, it either left itself open to co-optation or became irrelevant. For example, although R. D. Laing created a widespread furor in the 1960s, his ultimate inability to connect himself with any really radical social critique[40] left Laing's insights adrift on an existentialist sea. As a result his late work has tended to lapse into mysticism and triviality. Where Laing lost the thread, that other influential anti-psychiatry critic of the 1960s, Thomas Szasz, took it in the wrong direction. Szasz's criticism of psychiatric labelling and oppression[41] was grounded in a conception of individual liberty so devoid of connection to the real social roots of injustice as to become positively reactionary. From another angle, the radical psychiatry movement of the 1960s showed that it was possible to begin a radical social critique of mental health along Marxist lines.[42] Despite this beginning, however, the movement proved even more sterile than the Laingian. For one thing the radical psychiatrists shared the antipathy to theory endemic to the American Left. Such Marxism as they employed consequently tended to be vulgar and economistic, and could not comprehend the forms capitalist domination takes in its late period. This theoretical myopia, associated with a striking degree of psychological know-nothingism, left the radical psychiatrists unable to pay attention to the real subjective phenomena of emotional disturbance. Generally implacably hostile to Freud because of his sexism and class-bias, they refused to recognize the reality of what he discovered, and instead devoted themselves to the direct, unmediated connection between objective, socially-imposed oppression and the subjective hobblings of neurosis and psychosis. The psychiatric establishment, pragmatic if not profound, has always taken enough cognizance of the reality of emotional disturbance to win people's attention. The radical psychiatrists, on the other hand, became quixotically irrelevant and faded, the failure of their therapeutics joining with that of their politics.

Such is the spectacle of the American mental health industry. One is inclined to call it an unreassuring prospect. The good that has been done to particular individuals and families in need of care remains, to be sure. But it has to be weighed against the large-scale social effects wrought by the class of experts who administer these benefits. At this level one must conclude that the ultimate impact of the mental health industry is to increase alienation and false consciousness. It does so by the *content* of what it conveys, namely the myth of individual psychology and cure in the midst of a diseased society; and, more fundamentally, it does so by the *form* by which it conveys the myth, i.e. that of *expertise* itself: technocracy descending from above, like white gods coming from the skies to colonize the natives.

Alienation is a two-way process, affecting ruler as well as ruled. And loss of contact with the living historical root of their work has exacted a toll upon the mental health industry. A sense of stagnation reigns; the innovations seem to have fallen exhausted into the stifling embrace of bureaucracy. An empty formalism prevails at the center, while at the periphery the search for shibboleths resembles the parlor-psychology games widely sold at department stores. Meanwhile organic psychiatry has begun to rise again. Biological research has become the ticket to academic success and brain science is trumpeted as some kind of revolutionary advance. Most ominous has been a revival of the behemoth of psychosurgery, influential in the 1940s and 1950s, but dormant since. This time the state itself is giving its seal of approval, a Congressionally mandated commission having recently concluded that lobotomy might not only be helpful for certain supposedly pure psychiatric syndromes, but possibly useful as well for the control of 'impulsive aggressiveness', even extending to the case of such prisoners 'whose capacity to consent may be somewhat diminished'.[43]

But this chilling development – revealing as it does the potential for the totalitarian takeover of mind – reminds us once again of the essential dependency of mental health on the fortunes of capitalist society as a whole. It is therefore pointless to wring one's hands about the sad state of today's theory and practice without taking account of the dialectical opportunity this represents. If mental hygiene has near run its course, it is because capitalism is running out of excuses. The very encroachments of the state have created new pockets of resistance. As the boundary between public and private practice disappears, those with originality and spirit will have to figure out new combinations to realize the goals of the first wave of radical psychiatrists without relapsing into their shortsightedness. Already there are signs of stirring for a second wave. This has been spurred in part by the proletarianization of mental health workers resulting from the fact that while the state has largely taken over the field, it has also had to shift resources away from human-service programs in the face of the chronic crisis afflicting world capitalism. In such times as these, priorities have to be restored to the accumulation process, leaving the state's needs for legitimation undermanned. Mental health workers are feeling the economic squeeze while still being asked to perform their hygienic function. As a result a number are for the first time developing class-consciousness: some psychiatric residents having gone so far as to break with professionalism and strike.[44] Whether these beginnings will go anywhere is anybody's guess. But that they exist is indisputable. History will out, and has its surprises.

3 On the Medicalization of Deviance and Social Control

Peter Conrad

A man in Baltimore, arrested several times for exhibitionism, goes to a physician for a new drug, Depo-Provera, for treatment of his deviant behavior. A well-known surgeon in a southwestern American city performs a psychosurgical operation on a young man who is prone to violent outbursts. A child in California brought to a pediatric clinic because of his disruptive behavior in school is labeled hyperactive and prescribed Ritalin for his disorder. In an East Coast prison a man is given medication 'to alleviate his mood disorder' after a recent altercation with prison authorities. A chronically overweight Chicago housewife receives a surgical by-pass operation as treatment for her problem of obesity. Scientists in a New England medical center work on a million-dollar federal research grant to discover a heroin-blocking agent and 'cure' heroin addiction. In all these instances medical solutions are being sought for behavioral problems and social deviance. The medicalization of deviance and attendant medical social control is becoming increasingly prevalent in modern industrial societies.

Medical practitioners and medical treatment in our society usually are viewed as healing the sick and giving comfort to the afflicted. No doubt these are important aspects of medicine. In recent years the jurisdiction of the medical profession has expanded and has encompassed many problems that formerly were not defined as medical entities. Ivan Illich recently has termed this 'the medicalization of life'.[1] While there is much to be said for this viewpoint – e.g. the medicalization of pregnancy and childbirth, contraception, diet, exercise, child development norms, etc. – my concern here is more limited and specific. My interest focuses on the medicalization of deviant behavior: the defining and labeling of deviant behavior as a medical problem, an illness, and mandating the medical profession to provide some type of treatment for it. Concomitant with this is the growing utilization of medicine as an agent of social control, typically as medical intervention. Medical intervention as social control seeks to limit, modify, regulate, isolate or eliminate socially defined deviant behavior, *with medical means and in the name of health*.[2] This chapter examines sociologically the emergence and development of medicalization and medical control especially in the U.S.A. where it is most pronounced. It presents an analysis of the transformation of deviance from *badness to sickness* and the adoption of a medical model of behavior.

Before beginning an analysis of medicalization it is important to present two general sociological notions that pertain to the argument presented here. These include the social construction of illness and the relationship of illness and deviance.

The social construction of illness. What are disease and illness? On the face of it they seem rather straightforward concepts. A commonsense viewpoint might see disease as something that exists 'out there', apart even from the human body, that may enter the body and do harm: ideas of avoiding viruses, germs and other 'diseases' follow from this view. A systematized variant of a commonsense view might be that disease is 'a specific destructive process in an organism, with specific causes and specific symptoms'.[3] Sometimes disease is seen simply as a departure from health. Illness, if differentiated from disease at all, is taken as the condition of being diseased or, more commonly, the state of being sick. Yet, as I will argue, disease and illness are highly complex entities, far more problematic than these commonsense views indicate. It is not my goal here to settle a longstanding academic controversy on the nature of disease and illness,[4] but rather to sensitize the reader to a number of approaches and to some characteristics of illness designations.

A positivist conception of illness is most similar to the commonsense view. Illness is the presence of disease in an organism that inhibits the functioning, or 'well working' in Leon Kass's terms,[5] of the physiological organs (in a most inclusive sense) of the organism. This strict and limiting definition includes only malfunctioning organs as diseases. However, there is an implicit assumption of the existence of some norm of functioning or well working that can be measured against and that this normal condition will be recognizable by the medical observer. One need only think about the controversies surrounding tonsils and tonsillectomies to realize that well functioning of organs is a problematic concept in itself. And besides, does such a notion limiting illness and disease to organ malfunctioning include undiscovered diseases or organ changes that may be adaptations to an environment (e.g. the sickle cell trait)? By focusing only on 'objective' organ conditions, the positivists (at least in theory) delimit their concept of disease. It is important to point out that most of the difficulties that we term mental illness, especially the functional disorders, do not match this definition at all.

Others have argued that disease and illness are separate entities and can be analysed separately. Abram Feinstein 'conceptualizes disease in purely morphologic, physiologic, and chemical terms. What the physician observes directly in his dialogue (examination) that he terms *illness* consists of subjective sensations (symptoms) and certain findings (signs). The illness described is the result of the interaction of the disease with the host or person, emphasis being given to the mechanism by which disease develops or produces and is associated with the illness.'[6] According to this viewpoint disease is a physiological state and illness is a social state presumably caused by the disease. While the pathologist views the disease, the physician sees only the signs and symptoms of illness and infers disease. This allows, conceptually at least, for illnesses without diseases and diseases without illnesses. Such a body/social dichotomy has the advantage of permitting analysis on both the physiological and social levels.

In sharp contrast to the positivist viewpoint is the cultural relativist position: An entity or condition is a disease or illness only if it is recognized and defined as one by the culture. For example, in one South American Indian tribe, dyschromic spirochetosis, a disease characterized by colored spots appearing on the skin, was so common that those who did not have it were regarded as deviant and excluded from marriage.[7] Amongst the Papago Indians of the American Southwest obesity has a prevalence of nearly 100 per cent. Yet the Papago do not regard this condition as abnormal; in fact, they often bring babies whose development is normal by Western standards to the medical clinic and ask the physician what's wrong with their baby, why is he so skinny and sickly. To the Papago obesity is not an illness; by Western medical standards nearly all the Papago are ill. Which definition is more valid? Dubos has argued that a universal condition that is 'health' is a mirage and that health and illness are limited by cultural knowledge and conditions and adaptations to the environment.[8] Certainly such a relativist stance has some credence, perhaps especially with what we call mental illness, but is criticized for minimizing the organic-physiological nature of illness and disease. However, cultural relativists sensitize us to the variability in the interpretation and definition of physiological phenomena.

While all these approaches have some utility and validity in the contexts in which they are utilized, from a sociological perspective they miss a crucial aspect of illness: They take for granted how something becomes defined as an illness in the first place. Illness and diseases are human constructions; they do not exist without someone recognizing and defining them. There are processes that *we* term diseases, but that does not make them *a priori* diseases. As Peter Sedgwick points out, 'the blight that strikes corn or potatoes is a *human invention*, for if man wished to cultivate parasites (instead of corn or potatoes) there would be no "blight" but simply the necessary foddering of a parasite crop'.[9] An animal may be feebled, have parasites, or be in pain but that in no way means they are suffering from an illness.

Animals do not have diseases either, prior to the presence of man in a meaningful relation with them. A tiger may experience pain or feebleness from a variety of causes ... It may be infected by a germ, trodden by an elephant, scratched by another tiger, or subjected to the aging process of its own cells. It does not present itself as being *ill* (though it may present itself as highly distressed or uncomfortable) except in the eyes of the human observer who can discriminate illness from other sources of pain and enfeeblement. Outside the significance that man voluntarily attaches to certain conditions, *there are no illnesses or diseases in nature.*[10]

There are of course naturally occurring events, including infectious viruses, malignant growths, ruptures of tissues, unusual chromosome constellations, but these are not *ipso facto* illnesses. Without the social meaning that humans attach to them they do not constitute illnesses or disease. 'The fracture of a septuagenarian's femur has, within the world of nature, no more significance than the snapping of an autumn leaf from its twig: and the invasion of a human organism by cholera germs carries with it no more the stamp of "illness" than the souring of milk by other forms of bacteria.'[11] Hence, one could argue that biophysiological phenomena are what we use as a basis to label one condition or another as an illness or disease; the biophysiological phenomena are not in themselves illness or disease.

Illnesses are human judgments on conditions that exist in the natural world. They are essentially *social constructions* – hypothetical constructs of our own creation. The fact that there is high agreement on what constitutes an illness does not change this: The high degree of consensus on what 'objectively' is disease is not independent from the social consensus that constructs these 'facts'. For physical illness the consensus is so extensive and taken for granted that we are inclined to impute a reality independent of our agreement.[12]

As illnesses are social judgments, they are negative judgments.[13] An entity that is labeled an illness or disease is clearly considered undesirable. In the human world this is as true for tuberculosis and cancer as it is for mental illness and alcoholism. Biological aberration is neither necessary nor sufficient for something to be labeled an illness: a seven-foot basketball player is biologically abnormal but not ill. Early and late onset of puberty are both biologically deviant conditions yet only late puberty is viewed as evidence for physiological abnormalities and disorder (as 'developmental delays'). Nearly all functional mental disorders have no or at best questionable physiological evidence, yet they are defined and treated as diseases. In Western societies most illnesses are assumed to have some biophysiological or organic basis (and most do), but this is not a necessary condition for something to be defined as an illness. However, most physiological conditions that are found troublesome are defined as illnesses.

As Eliot Freidson observes, calling something an illness in human society has *consequences independent* of the biological condition of the organism.

... when a veterinarian diagnoses a cow's condition as an illness, he does not merely by his diagnosis change the cow's behavior: to the cow, illness remains an experienced biophysiological state, no more. But when a physician diagnoses a human's condition as illness, he changes the man's behavior by diagnosis; a social state is added to the biophysiological state by assigning the meaning of illness to disease.[14]

Think of the difference in consequences if a person's inability to function is attributed to laziness or to mononucleosis, seizures to demon possession or epilepsy, or drinking habits to moral weakness or alcholism. Medical diagnosis affects people's behavior, attitudes they take toward themselves, and attitudes others take toward them.

In summary, illness is a social construction based on human judgment of some condition in the world. In some fashion illness, like beauty, is in the eyes of the beholder. While it is partly based on current cultural conceptions of what disease is, and more often than not in Western society grounded in biophysiological phenomena, this social evaluative process is central rather than peripheral to the concept of illness and disease. It follows logically that both diagnosis (as systematized classifications) and treatments are founded on these social judgments; they cannot be separated. Just as there were profound consequences from the recognition of microorganisms as agents of 'disease' so are there consequences from recognizing illnesses as social judgments. Needless to add, the social construction of illness for behavioral deviancy is subject to more ambiguity and interpretation than manifestly biophysiological problems. In this light it is understandable that conditions defined as illness reflect the social values and general *weltanshauung* of a society.

Illness and deviance. As Talcott Parsons pointed out in his classic writings on the 'sick role', both crime and illness are designations for deviant behavior.[15] Parsons conceptualized illness as deviance primarily because of its threat to the stability of a social system through its impact on role performance. While both crime and illness are violations of norms (social and medical) and can be disruptive to social life, the attributions of cause are different. Deviance that is seen as *willful* tends to be defined as crime; when it is seen as *unwillful* it tends to be defined as illness. Since crime and illness are both designations of deviance it becomes necessary to distinguish between the two, especially with reference to the appropriate mechanisms of social control. It is in this regard that Parsons developed his notion of the sick role.

The social responses to crime and illness are different. The criminal is punished with the goal of altering his or her motivations toward conventionality; the sick person is treated with the goal of altering the conditions that prevent his or her conventionality. Parsons further argues that there exists for the sick a culturally available 'sick role' that serves to conditionally legitimate the deviance of illness and to channel the sick into the reintegrating doctor-patient relationship, therefore minimizing its disruptiveness to the group or society. The sick role has four components, two exemptions from normal responsibilities and two new obligations. First, the sick person is exempted from normal responsibilities, at least to the extent necessary to 'get well'. Second, the individual is not held responsible for his or her condition and cannot be expected to recover by an act of will. Third, the person must recognize that being ill is an inherently undesirable state, and must want to recover. Fourth, the sick person is obligated to seek and cooperate with a competent treatment agent (usually a physician).[16] Implicit in the sick role is the notion that medicine is an institution of social control. As legitimater of the sick role and as healer returning the sick to conventional social roles, the physician functions as a social control agent.

In the light of the discussion here, it is significant to note that since crime and illness are both socially constructed designations for deviance, it should not be surprising that there has been a fluidity between designations of crime deviations and illness deviations. One of the major concerns of this chapter is exploring the factors contributing to the change from moral-criminal definitions of deviance to medical ones. It is to this medicalization of deviance we now turn.

The medicalization of deviance

Conceptions of deviant behavior change and agencies mandated to control deviance shift also. Historically there have been great transformations in the definition of deviance – from religious to moral to state to medical-scientific. Emile Durkheim noted in *The Division of Labor in Society* that as societies develop from simple to more complex, sanctions for deviance change from repressive to restitutive or, put another way, from punishment to treatment or rehabilitation.[17] Along with the change in sanctions and social control agent there is a corresponding change in definition or conceptualization of deviant behavior. For example, deviant drinking (what we call alcoholism) has been defined as sin, moral weakness, crime and, most recently, illness. Nicholas Kitterie, from a legal standpoint, has called this change the devestment of criminal justice and the coming of the therapeutic state.[18] Philip Rieff, in his sociological study of the impact of Freudian thought, terms it the triumph of the therapeutic.[19]

In modern industrial society there has been a substantial growth in the prestige, dominance, and jurisdiction of the medical profession. Until the last century, physicians were relatively unorganized, inconsistently trained, poorly paid, and limited in their therapeutic techniques and abilities. Eminent American physician Dr Lawrence J. Henderson observed that 'somewhere between 1910 and 1912 in this country, a random patient, with a random disease, consulting a doctor chosen at random had, for the first time in the history of mankind, a better than fifty-fifty chance of profiting from the encounter'.[20] With the apparent success of medicine in controlling communicable disease,[21] the growth of scientific biomedicine, the regulation of medical education and licensing, and the political organization and lobbying of the American Medical Association, the prestige of the medical profession has increased. The medical profession dominates the organization of health care and has a virtual monopoly on anything that is defined as medical treatment, especially in terms of what constitutes 'illness' and what is appropriate medical intervention. As Freidson has pointed out, 'The medical profession has first claim to jurisdiction over the label illness and *anything* to which it may be attached, irrespective of its capacity to deal with it effectively.'[22] Reiff contends that the hospital has replaced the church and parliament as the symbolic center of Western society.[23] While Durkheim did not predict this medicalization, perhaps in part because medicine of his time was not the scientific, prestigious, and dominant profession of today, it is clear that medicine is the central restitutive agent in our society.

As treatment rather than punishment becomes the preferred sanction for deviance, an increasing amount of behavior is conceptualized as illness in a medical framework. As noted above, this is not unexpected as medicine always functioned as an agent of social control, especially in attempting to 'normalize' illness and return people to their functioning capacity in society. Public health and psychiatry have long been concerned with social behavior and have traditionally functioned as agents of control.[24] What is significant, however, is the expansion of the sphere where medicine now functions as an agent of social control. In the wake of a general humanitarian trend, the success and prestige of modern biomedicine, the increasing acceptance of deterministic social and medical concepts, the technological growth of the twentieth century, and the diminution of religion as a viable agent of control, more and more deviant behavior has come into the province of medicine. With these developments has come a change of the conception of deviance; much deviance that was badness (i.e. sinful or criminal) is now sickness. While some forms of deviant behavior are more completely medicalized than others (e.g. mental illness), recent work has pointed to a considerable variety of deviance that has been treated with medical jurisdiction: alcoholism, drug addiction, hyperactive children, suicide, obesity, crime, violence, child abuse, learning problems, amongst others.[25] Concomitant with medicalization has been a change in imputed responsibility for deviance: with badness the deviant was considered responsible for the behavior, with sickness he or she is not, or at least responsibility is diminished. The social response to deviance is 'therapeutic' rather than punitive.[26]

A number of social factors underlie the medicalization of deviance. As psychiatric critic Thomas Szasz has observed:

> With the transformation of the religious perspective of man into the scientific, and in particular the psychiatric, which became fully articulated during the nineteenth century, there occurred a radical shift in emphasis away from viewing man as a *responsible agent acting in and on the world* and toward viewing him *as a responsive organism being acted upon* by biological and social 'forces'.[27]

This is exemplified by the diffusion of Freudian thought which, since the 1920s, has had a significant impact on the treatment of deviance, the distribution of stigma, and the incidence of penal sanctions. Kitterie, focusing on decriminalization, contends that the foundation of the therapeutic state is in determinist criminology, that it stems from the *parens patrie* power of the state (the state's right to help those who are deemed unable to help themselves), and dates its origin with the development of juvenile justice at the turn of the century.[28] Others have pointed out that the strength of informal sanctions is declining because of the increase in geographical mobility and the decrease in strength of traditional status groups (e.g. the family), and that medicalization offers a substitute method for controlling deviance.[29] The success of medicine in certain areas (e.g. infectious disease) had led to rising expectations of what medicine can accomplish. Clearly, the increasing acceptance and dominance of a scientific world-view and the increase in status and power of the medical profession have contributed significantly to medicalization.

While the aforementioned conditions created a climate for medicalization and underlie presentday changes in deviance designations, it is important to draw out more specifically conditions necessary to medicalize deviant behavior in contemporary society. I will rely primarily on the example with which I am most familiar, hyperactivity in children, to outline these conditions. When possible I will make references to other forms of deviance for comparison and illustration.

Hyperactivity is a good example to use as it is a relatively recent medical diagnostic category. It was first described by Maurice Laufer and his associates as the 'hyperkinetic impulse disorder' in 1957, although the roots of its 'discovery' can be traced to the 1930s.[30] It is considered a childhood behavior disorder with an assumed organic basis, usually medically labeled as 'Hyperactive Syndrome' or 'Minimal Brain Dysfunction', and treated with stimulant medications. Symptoms of hyperactivity include extreme excess of motor activity, inattentiveness, restlessness, fidgetiness, impulsivity, mood swings, difficulties in school and aggressive-like behaviors. In the U.S.A. it is considered the single most common child psychiatric problem and is commonly treated by family pediatricians, with an estimated prevalence of 3 per cent to 10 per cent of elementary school children.

The conditions for the medicalization of deviance

A behavior or set of behaviors must be defined as deviant and as a problem in need of remedy by some segment of society. As sociologists of the labeling/societal reaction persuasion have pointed out in recent decades, before 'deviant behavior' can exist, the behavior must be socially defined as deviant.[31] Many forms of behavior have been defined as deviant in one society or era and not in another; deviance is in its essence a social definition. Like illness, it is a social construction. Hence, before 'deviance' can be medicalized, behavior must be defined and recognized as deviant. Hyperactive-type behavior surely existed before Laufer *et al.*'s diagnostic description, and it is likely that it was at least sometimes considered deviant behavior. Certainly restlessness, extreme activity, not paying attention and not sitting still were defined as deviant behavior in school classrooms and in many family settings.

In addition to being defined as deviant, some persons in society, generally with more social power than the deviant, must view the behavior as a problem. Not all forms of behavior defined by some as deviance are construed as problems in need of remedies; for example, defiance of 'blue laws', cohabitation, some forms of sexual deviance (e.g. swinging), and gambling are usually not seen as in need of remedy. Homosexuality is still defined as deviance in our society, but is increasingly not seen as a problem in need of remedy (e.g. less enforcement of 'crimes against nature' laws and the 1973 American Psychiatric Association resolution not to define it as an illness). It is necessary that those who define the deviance as in need of remedy have the power to implement their definitions. For example, if some students defined price-fixing and profiteering among corporate executives as deviance and a problem in need of remedy, they ordinarily would not have the power to implement their definitions of the situation.

When *previous or traditional forms of social control are seen as inefficient or unacceptable*, it is likely that medical controls will appear. Forms and methods of social control change. Those regarded as mentally ill were at various times chained, bled, locked in wards, given psychotherapy or medicated, all with the similar goal: to control their behavior and minimize the disruptiveness of their deviance on society. Criminals have been pilloried, executed, imprisoned, and most recently behavior modified in an attempt to minimize and control their deviant behavior. Religion was once the main source of social control with confessions, excommunications and inquisitions. For nearly four hundred years the state has been the most important administrator of social control. In modern society medicine is becoming an increasingly powerful and common form of social control, especially in terms of psychotherapy, drugs and surgery. The shift from religious to state to medical social control is often depicted as a humanitarian modernization of the social control networks of society but probably better reflects the changes in the *zeitgeist* rather than any progressive improvement.

Medicalization occurs when traditional or previous forms of social control are no longer efficient or acceptable. There have probably been some effective 'traditional' forms of social control for overactive or restless behavior in schoolchildren. The oldfashioned, highly disciplined schoolroom with a hickory stick perhaps was sufficient control for some children.[32] If this was unsuccessful, the children could be asked not to attend school, and they could go to work. While there is still some corporal punishment in schools, it is no longer a major form of social control. It is relatively difficult to expel an elementary school child from school; certainly there is no work for a nine-year-old reject. On the other hand, children may no longer drop out of school until a certain age (14 to 16 in most states), so they somehow must remain in school. Additionally there is great pressure to stay in school – certainly a high school diploma is seen as a minimal necessity for most future employment. As the traditional social controls in schools have become unacceptable (many of them were not efficient either) through the general liberalization of the classroom experience, the need for newer, more 'liberal', forms of social controls arose. Many of these, although sometimes helpful, have not been very efficient as forms of classroom social control: tracking, guidance counseling, psychotherapy for children, or even sending the child to a 'quiet room'. While there is certainly no 'conspiracy' involved, these changes in the school (perhaps coupled with more 'permissive' childrearing in the family) created conditions that were more conducive to the acceptance of new forms of control. Witness the popularity of special classes and behavior modification in the modern elementary classroom, as well as the identification and treatment (with medications) of hyperactive children.

While this is not the place to discuss classroom control, I use this example to point out that methods of acceptable social control change and if more efficient forms of control become available they may be adopted. The problem of disruptive children in elementary school classrooms has probably always existed, only our manners for dealing with it are new. Treatments, such as behavior modification and medication, rather than punishments are more acceptable in our society.

For deviance to be medicalized, *some medical form of social control needs to be available.* If treatment rather than punishment is more acceptable in our society, the major source of treatment expertise is the medical profession and the related medico-technological research complex. Clearly, medical control *qua* treatment cannot replace or complement existing or traditional forms of social control unless forms of medical social control are available. At the present time, these controls usually take the form of psychoactive medications, surgical procedures and more vaguely genetic engineering. With a vast medical technology industry including powerful pharmaceutical corporations engaged in research, new discoveries in genetics, and modern psychosurgical procedures, new forms of medical controls (as treatments) are often discovered. Some of these medical controls themselves may not be acceptable to society, others are. Some like methadone are seen as panaceas.

Charles Bradley observed in 1937 that recently invented amphetamine drugs had a spectacular 'paradoxical' effect in altering the behavior of school children who exhibited behavior disorders or learning difficulties.[33] For the next twenty years, despite a few concurring reports, this remained a rather esoteric medical finding. Following the publication of Laufer *et al.*'s description of the hyperactive impulse disorder and increased promotion by the pharmaceutical industry, hyperactivity and its treatment with stimulant medications became well known, identified and treated. By the 1970s hyperactivity was a part of everyday vocabulary and approximately 250,000–400,000 American children were being treated for it.

It is my judgment that in our modern and technological society, virtually all new forms of social control will be either medical or some other psychotechnology such as behavior modification. These forms of control are, if nothing else, generally more efficient than other forms of control and may be implemented in the name of humanitarian progress. For example, research has shown that in 60 to 70 per cent of children diagnosed as hyperactive there is 'improvement', that is behavior becomes more socially acceptable. The majority of such controls are administered as medical treatments: psychosurgery for violent behavior, antibuse for alcoholism, stimulant medication for hyperactive children, psychoactive drugs for mental disorder, methadone for drug addiction, genetic screening for XYY males, and most recently Depo-Provera for sexual obsessions. The discovery of a medical mechanism of control may considerably predate the actual medicalization of deviance; hyperactivity was not named until two decades after the medical form of control was discovered. Availability of medical control mechanism is necessary though not sufficient for medicalization to occur.

Another factor that seems to be necessary, at least in Western societies, for medicalization *is the existence of some ambiguous organic data as to the source of the problem*. Rarely have scientists discovered clear direct 'causes' for deviant behavior, or for that matter, for any behavior. Social scientists usually present 'causal' explanations in terms of variables, correlations, contingencies, or conditions which will increase the probability of certain forms of behavior. Such research is usually *post facto* and retrospective, and while controls are used to validate findings, social scientific predication of individual behavior is rather primitive and unreliable.

In general, organic or physiological factors are more specific and thought to yield better predictions than social factors. This may in part be due to the success of discovering etiologic specificity with communicable diseases. Yet there are often gray areas with physiological causal explanations also. This is especially true in inferring causal connections from physiological variables to certain forms of behavior. The data or the connections to behavior are usually ambiguous. Sometimes organic or physiological factors are found as correlates of certain behavior. For example, an extra Y chromosome has been found in a statistically significant number of men in institutions for the criminally insane;[34] abnormal EEGs in some persons who have committed violent acts; 'soft neurological signs' in hyperactive children. These physiological correlates then become etiological explanations: the deviant behavior is purported to be 'caused' by the organic difficulty.

In other cases the ambiguous organic data are largely dependent on an organic treatment that is at least somewhat successful: heroin addiction and methadone, sociopathic persons and epinephrine, and violence and psychosurgery. The organic component is assumed from the treatment. While this is not the place to evaluate critically each of these findings or treatments, they each present some evidence, however ambiguous, for a biophysiological component as a cause for deviant behavior.

Hyperactivity again can serve as an example. There are numerous organic biophysiological theories for hyperactivity etiology, all of which have some evidence: for example, brain injury, minimal brain dysfunction, prenatal or perinatal difficulties, innate temperament, genetic disorder, lead poisoning, and food additives in the diet all have been postulated as causes of hyperactivity. Each of these theories has some supporting data, although none is unequivocal; a recent review has found the data for organicity to be wanting.[35] The actual evidence used to make a diagnosis is also ambiguous and open to various interpretations; many findings used to postulate organic dysfunction are found also in non-hyperactive children, although usually with less frequency. My own research at a pediatric diagnostic clinic leads me to conclude that hyperactivity as a diagnosis is as much a product of the social process in which the medical reality is constructed as it is a product of any objective physiological reality.[36] The major point is not that there is no organic component to hyperactivity (the evidence is far from complete) but rather that for deviance to be medicalized there must be data from which organicity can be hypothesized.

Before something can be medicalized, it is essential for *the medical profession to accept the deviant behavior within their jurisdiction.* Medicalization is not possible without the complicity or willingness of at least some part of the medical profession. Physicians, as the legitimate sources of medical definitions, are necessary to define an entity as within the medical sphere and virtually have a monopoly of any knowledge or treatment that relates to the dysfunctioning of the physical body. It may be only a small segment of the profession that views the deviance within the medical sphere, as for example with violence, but it is necessary that some physicians accept it within their jurisdiction. The degree of specialization in the profession, the flexible boundaries of medicine, and the availability of research monies facilitate the expansion of medical jurisdiction.

Often there are medical professionals who act as entrepreneurs for medicalization. With hyperactivity, the basic research on diagnosis and treatment was conducted by about a dozen physicians and behavioral scientists (with colleagues). Of this group, three or four (and later others) published a number of papers promoting hyperactivity, exhorting the usefulness of medical treatment, and advocating the identification and treatment of hyperactive children. For whatever professional, scientific or other reasons, such medical enterprise facilitates medicalization.

The medicalization of hyperactivity and drug addiction were both symbolically approved by blue ribbon professional investigative committees. For hyperactivity this approval came in a report submitted to the Department of Health, Education and Welfare's Office of Child Development in 1971; for drug addiction it was a 1960 report of the Joint Committee of the American Bar Association and American Medical Association. The recent report of a commission mandated by the Department of Health, Education and Welfare endorsing psychosurgery as having 'potential merit' without 'excessive' risks, is a further example of this.[37] Such prestigious professional and government approval increases the acceptance of deviant behavior as a legitimate medical problem.

As medicalization affects society beyond the medical profession and the deviants, it is also affected by society. I would suggest the greater the benefit of medicalization to established institutions, the more likely it is to occur. This can be illustrated with several case examples. In the 1960s heroin addiction and, perhaps more specifically, crime allegedly by addicts who needed increasing resources to maintain their addiction, became a major social concern. Traditional forms of control such as prison and peer self-help groups had only limited success, as well as being overburdened and relatively expensive. Methadone maintenance as a treatment for heroin addiction – ironically by substituting one addiction for another – was in many ways a less expensive, simpler and more efficient form of control. Numerous established institutions benefited from this medicalization and hence supported it; the courts and prisons reduced their contact with addicts;

the police and community, at least in theory, had a little less 'drug connected' crime with which to contend; the hospital and mental health facilities could now treat addicts by simpler and quicker means; and pharmaceutical corporations could profit from methadone manufacture.

Restless, fidgety children, who do not sit still or pay attention in school and who are often disruptive and difficult to manage at home, have probably always been with us. However, medicalizing hyperactivity is beneficial to important established institutions. Schools now have an effective means of reducing the disruptiveness of such children; families too are less disrupted and parents need not feel guilt as the cause is considered to be organic; pharmaceutical companies who have heavily promoted stimulant medical treatment for hyperactivity, have managed a substantial profit – reportedly $13 million from Ritalin in 1970 alone – from their manufacture, and physicians themselves have another means of 'helping' distressed families with their internal problems.

A further word should be added about the pharmaceutical corporations. They are frequently entrepreneurs for medicalization: a classic example has been the promotion of Valium, Librium and other tranquilizers for such common problems as anxiety, nervousness, 'bluesiness', and general malaise. The pharmaceutical industry spends over $1 billion per year for promotion of prescription drugs largely to physicians, fully 25 per cent of the total sales dollars. And they are successful. In 1974, 59,500,000 Valium prescriptions were filled in America, making Valium the best selling prescription drug in the country.[38] The drug industry has been the number one or number two profitable industry in the United States for nearly two decades.

When a certain definition and treatment of deviance becomes institutionalized, vested interests develop to maintain that definition. Research monies, treatment centers, and even entire bureaucratic organizations organize around the treatment of deviance. Harrison Trice and Paul Roman describe 'the alcoholism industry' as 'those who design and implement programs for the prevention and treatment of problem drinking, as well as those who attempt to obtain financial support for efforts to deal with these problems'.[39] Such 'industries', which are often directly tied to the medical profession, lobby for and promote their particular conception and treatment of deviance.

In an age when science and scientific thinking reign supreme, any explanation of etiology or treatment must, to have credence with the medical profession and much of the public, be presented in scientific form. I suspect the greater the acceptance of this explanation, especially by professionals and legislators, the more likely behavior is to be medicalized. This is especially true in the converse: if a proposed scientific explanation is not accepted or is viewed as esoteric or extreme, medicalization is unlikely. Theories or treatments out of the medical mainstream are often treated with great skepticism, whether they concern the relationship of vitamin C and the common cold, megavitamin therapy and mental illness, or food additives and hyperactivity.

While the predominant trend has been the medicalization of deviance, an instructive example of *demedicalization* exists. Homosexuality, which was largely medicalized as psychiatric illness, has recently been at least symbolically demedicalized. The official demedicalization came at the December 1973 American Psychiatric Association convention when the delegates voted that it was no longer to be considered an illness. While the factors that led to this decision are complex, the precipitating agent was the politicization of the issue by persons in the 'gay liberation' movement. In light of the discussion above, it is insightful to note that homosexuality never had significant organic data supporting the illness definition,[40] and medical treatment was not particularly successful. It is doubtful that demedicalization would have occurred had there been reasonably compelling organic data and/or a successful treatment, for example as exists with epilepsy. While few medicalized deviant groups have organized and politicized the adoption of illness designations, the case of homosexuality clearly points up the political nature of adopting or relinquishing the medical model of deviant behavior.

Medicalization in society

As I have argued, the medicalization of deviance and social control is increasing and is rooted in the development of modern technological societies. Assuredly medicalization is not limited to the United States. Medicalized approaches are common in Western Europe and undoubtedly will spread as the influence of Western biomedicine and the multinational pharmaceutical industry expands throughout the world. Already, although from somewhat different reasons, the medicalization of political dissidents as mentally ill is frequent in the Soviet Union and perhaps in other countries as well.[41]

It is fair to ask, what does this all mean? Why should there be any concern about the medicalization of deviance? While a full discussion of this is beyond the scope of this chapter, it is important to point out some of the more salient consequences of medicalization. Beyond the now obvious and most significant observation that medical definitions of deviance *remove responsibility* for behavior from the individual, there are other effects of medicalization. First is the seemingly endless expansion of the jurisdiction of medicine, regardless of its ability to deal adequately with a problem. This is fueled by a powerful, profitable and expansionary pharmaceutical industry and a growing interconnection between medicine and government. Second is the assumed moral neutrality of medicine. Medicine is influenced by the moral order of society – witness the nineteenth-century diagnosis and treatment for the disease of masturbation – yet medical language of disease and treatment is assumed to be morally neutral. It is not and the technological-scientific vocabulary of medicine often obfuscates this fact. Medicine reflects the moral order: otherwise why is heroin addiction a disease and not coffee addiction? Third, medicalization professionalizes human and social problems and delegates medical experts to handle them. There is a dominance and hegemony of medical definitions: they are often taken as the last scientific word. By medicalizing deviance we virtually remove it from the realm of public discussion and put it on a plane where only experts can discuss it. Fourth, medical social control utilizes powerful and sometimes non-reversible methods to 'treat' deviant behavior. These technological social control mechanisms, be they psychoactive drugs, surgery or genetic intervention, generally support the *status quo* of society. Fifth, medicalization individualizes human difficulties. By focusing on the individual's internal environment it largely ignores or minimizes the social nature of human behavior. As Irving Zola has noted, 'by locating the source and treatment of problems in individuals, other levels of intervention are closed'.[42] While this aligns well with the individualistic ethic of Western culture, it distorts reality and allows for social control in the name of health.

4 Towards a Critical History of the Psychiatric Profession

Andy Treacher and Geoff Baruch

Our concern in this chapter is to explore one major issue – the dominant role that the psychiatric profession plays within the mental health industry in Britain. Kovel in his chapter characterizes the American situation as bewildering and complex, but we would contend that although the British scene is becoming more complex, and there are the beginnings of a consumerist trend (exemplified by the growth of the encounter group movement and by many different types of self-help group), there remains a striking uniformity in the way that the majority of patients are processed by the system.

To many of our readers this contention may appear to be sheer dogmatism – surely important innovations are being made in many fields; family therapy is emerging as a new approach, most professionals within the area are better trained and more sophisticated, etc., etc. We would not dismiss such arguments out of hand, but we would insist that such changes are merely 'first-order' ones.[1] To argue that changes are occurring is a bit like arguing that because we are now playing musical chairs to a new tune, some profound change has occurred; clearly, for 'change' to occur in any profound sense, we would have to play an entirely new game.

But to extend our analogy still further, we would argue that not only are the game and even the tune still the same, the bandmasters are the same, too. In the British situation the bandmasters are, of course, psychiatrists. They retain, as a result of an historical victory which they won in the nineteenth century, a position of professional dominance which has not been effectively challenged by any other professional group. Eysenck's challenge to the profession, beginning with his attack on its psychoanalytic wing[2] and culminating in his challenge to the whole profession,[3] may have ruffled a few feathers but it is clear that the profession is not prepared to concede any of its powers. Nigel Goldie's fascinating study of the relationship between psychiatrists, social workers and clinical psychologists should be read by anybody who has illusions about this. As Goldie clearly shows, there is an essential hypocrisy involved in the working relationships between these three disciplines. In the final analysis the psychiatrist can claim that he is ultimately responsible for any crucial decisions that are to be made in relation to a patient whose care may have been initially delegated to other professionals.[4]

Goldie has also explored the role of 'eclecticism' in maintaining the professional dominance of psychiatry. He argues that it is precisely because the profession adheres to an eclectic approach that it cannot be challenged at a theoretical or ideological level. Typically any challenge that is made is absorbed rather than resisted, because the best tactical defence to any challenge is not a counter-challenge but a move which effectively defuses the attack.[5]

Anthony Clare's recent much-quoted book *Psychiatry in Dissent* is a good example of this type of approach. After enthusiastically demolishing other possible models of mental disorder Clare spells out his own position in the following terms:

I have made no mention of the so-called 'medical model' . . . The medical model is an evolving one in which scientific methods of observation, description, and differentiation are employed, in which an illness is conceptualized as a 'process that moves from the recognition and palliation of symptoms to the characterisation of a specific disease in which the etiology and pathogenesis are known and the treatment is rational and specific'. Such a process may take years, centuries even, and while many medical conditions have moved to the final stages of such understanding, others are still at various points along the way.[6]

This definition is, of course, very traditional and is largely indistinguishable from those of Lord, Mapother, Henderson, Lewis and many other influential psychiatrists who have explored the subject during the past fifty years. However, Clare is obviously a little more sophisticated than this – he writes, after all, in an era when even medical students receive some instruction in 'behavioural science'. He therefore appears rather dissatisfied with his first stab at a definition since he adds a rider which modifies it considerably:

The medical model does not envisage disease as something which 'happens' to a person independently of any action he may take . . . Medical diseases do not exist independently of the people who are sick. The medical model, in short, takes into account not merely the symptoms, syndrome, or disease but the person who suffers, his personal and social situation, his biological, psychological, and social status. The medical model, as applied to psychiatry, embodies the basic principle that every illness is the product of two factors – of environment working on the organism.[7]

Reading between the lines of Clare's argument, one can see that his model is designed to overarch all other approaches. As he says himself, 'it can be seen that the variety of ideological positions within psychiatry, the biological, the dynamic, the social, the behavioural, represent different emphases'. But Clare insists that if psychiatry is to progress, psychiatrists must continue to be eclectic. Psychiatrists must avoid giving their allegiance to any one model and avoid being dogmatic.

Clare's approach is, of course, very appealing to those who wallow in the various forms of empiricist anti-intellectualism which dominate thinking in the arena of mental health. This is why Clare is such a popular figure. His eminent reasonableness and apparent lack of dogma appeals to the British mind with its ingrained enthusiasm for compromise, for making do and mending. However, it should be pointed out that, as with all people who pretend to eschew dogmatism, Clare is himself clearly dogmatic in insisting that eclecticism is the only way forward.

In practice Clare's espoused theoretical position amounts to little more than a smokescreen for exerting the hegemony of the psychiatric profession, since it is clear from his book that he feels only a suitably trained psychiatrist is capable of taking the prime responsibility for the treatment of the mentally disordered. He is too subtle to spell this out directly, but when he comes to discuss the anatomy of the ideal psychiatrist he is really discussing the type of professional who can be expected to take such responsibility for the treatment of the mentally disordered.

Clare's ideal psychiatrist is a unique blend of virtue and knowledge, since he combines ' "the scientific attitudes of the sceptic with a powerful impressive personality and a profound existential faith". He is someone with a solid foundation in medicine, the biological and behavioural sciences, who is able to cope with the intellectual isolation implicit in such a critical eclecticism.' In practice Clare's view is little different from the position adopted by the newly founded Royal College of Psychiatrists. In 1973, the College submitted a memorandum to the D.H.S.S. expressing its views on the possible future role of psychological services within the N.H.S. The memorandum baldly states: 'It is recognized that there is a school of thought which denies the con-

cept of mental illness and considers that the symptoms hitherto classified as mental illness, mental disorder, tensions, psychoses, personality
disorders, etc., should be regarded as psychological behavioural mal-
adjustments and should be treated outside the medical orbit. These
views are not acceptable to the College'.[8]

Such a bald statement as this is clearly designed to protect the professional interests of psychiatrists; but is Clare's sophisticated view
any less a defence of the psychiatrist's hegemony? We would argue
that Clare's position remains basically reductionist – illnesses may
have psychological and sociological dimensions which must be 'taken
into account' (to use Clare's nebulous term), but their biological core
is primary and requires the skills that only the medically trained can
provide.

As we have already insisted, Clare has provided us with no new
insights largely because he has never broken with a tradition that has
a long heritage within British psychiatry. David Will has recently
pointed out[9] that this tradition has – despite its apparent espousal of
psychological approaches to mental disorder – proved antipathetic to
the development of psychotherapy, which is merely construed as one
approach among many others.

In Clare's model we are offered a view of the psychiatrist as master
detective – a veritable Sherlock Holmes who takes into account all
the myriad aspects of the patient, by drawing on every known science
which has relevance to human behaviour. After due accountancy a
treatment is usually devised which, if we are to take Clare's criticisms
of our own position seriously,[10] will most probably be a phenothiazine
(which, of course, only a psychiatrist can prescribe).

No doubt Clare will protest that this is a caricature of his model,
but we would insist that it is logical for a therapist with such an
eclectic and positivistic stance as Clare to end up prescribing drugs as
the main form of treatment. In doing so he of course operates within
a centuries-old tradition – medical men have always, as Ackernecht[11]
has clearly demonstrated, pursued panaceas, 'magic bullets', or indeed
bromides, with relentless devotion. In doing so, they have deluded us
into thinking that there are simple technological solutions to problems
which are endemic to the society in which we live. In this chapter we
will try to estimate the psychiatric profession's role in contributing to
this process of delusion-making, but before starting this discussion in
earnest it is necessary to return briefly to the point made by Will.

Will, in attacking the Meyerian tradition in which Clare operates, is a protagonist on behalf of psychoanalysis – he sees it as a liberating form of therapy which needs to be more widely adopted by the profession. But we would argue that such a position is as problematic as Clare's since it refuses to analyse the role of psychoanalysis itself. Kovel, Scull and many others have viewed psychoanalysis far more critically – they note that where psychoanalysis has become institutionalized (particularly within medicine), it has become a reactionary force. The underlying reductionism and determinism of Freud's model meant that it had immediate appeal to certain sections of the psychiatric profession who absorbed it without difficulty. But, needless to say, the more traditional and reactionary sections of the profession who sought to base psychiatry on the natural sciences (and particularly genetics) have always attempted to prevent Freudianism from obtaining a base within the profession. For them Freud's concentration on the necessity for self-analysis was anathema. Psychoanalysis' comparatively shallow roots within the British psychiatric profession is a tribute to the overall conservatism of the profession, but it is important to stress that from its inception psychoanalysis was dominated by sections of the medical profession.

David Smail, a leading clinical psychologist, has recently commented on the dual form of professional dominance that has been exerted by the medical profession in this respect. Reviewing the situation at the time when the N.H.S. was formed, he comments:

> Clinical psychologists were dwarfed by a medical guild whose powers, self-determination and freedom of action must be almost unique – the state of psychological knowledge ... did not permit psychologists to adopt anything but a secondary role. The physical methods of treatments appropriate to so-called mental illness obviously necessitated possession of a medical degree, and non-physical methods stemming, in this country, largely from the psycho-analytic school could only be practised by people (most usually doctors) who had undergone a lengthy and expensive initiation ceremony. In other words, the licence to practise treatment was based on a system where authority was accorded to would-be healers on the basis of membership of the appropriate (medical) club rather than on the basis of a scientifically demonstrable ability to assist psychological change. Above all, psychologists in the National Health Service were, and still are, prevented from direct involvement with patients by statutory constraints.[12]

The almost exclusive alignment of psychoanalysis with the medical profession in Britain contributed to its demise as a source of radical ideas. A single institution, the Tavistock Clinic, has played a quite disproportionate role in shaping the development of the psycho-analytic tradition, so that the British scene has lacked the variegated features of the American. This has resulted in an orthodoxy and conservatism which has survived the exciting but largely ephemeral work of Laing, Cooper and a number of other psychiatrists who broke away from the fold in the 1960s.

In order to understand the deep conservatism of British psychiatry as a whole, it is necessary to probe deeply into the history of the profession. Needless to say, commentators like Clare and Wing do not seriously examine historical issues in their accounts of the contemporary state of psychiatry; if they did so, they would uncover many uncomfortable issues which would undermine the assumptions from which they operate. Fortunately, Andrew Scull and David Ewins in their independent researches have recently provided us with a series of insights into the history of the psychiatric profession. At this point, our account therefore turns away from the contemporary scene to investigate the origins of psychiatry's position of dominance.

Scull in his work [13] has set himself one major task – to explain how a segment of the medical profession came to 'capture control over insanity'. The very words that Scull uses to describe his task indicate how sharply he breaks with the traditional presentation of the history of psychiatry in the nineteenth century. Usually the history is presented in a totally bland way: once upon a time some enlightened doctors set about the reform of an archaic and exploitative system of madhouses, workhouses, etc., in which the mad were cruelly treated. In doing so, they created our modern hospital system, which symbolizes the scientific and humane approach to the treatment of the mentally disordered. Interestingly, such accounts are often written by psychiatrists themselves, so there is always the uneasy suspicion that history is being distorted in order to justify the current dominance of the profession. The British psychiatrist, J. K. Wing, in his book *Reasoning about Madness* [14] provides us with the most recent example of this genre. His account of the impact of moral treatment on the asylums in Britain is particularly derisory as it totally ignores both the controversial nature of such methods and the special care that the medical profession took to establish (quite spuriously, as Scull demonstrates) that only members of the medical profession were capable of supervising them.

Fortunately Scull, through his extensive use of primary source material, provides us with a far more convincing account of developments within psychiatry in this crucial period. However, unlike Wing, he views the takeover bid by the psychiatric profession in a much broader context – as the following quotation reveals:

> In the first place one should notice that the shift in locus of responsibility for lunatics from the family and the local community to a group of trained professionals ... is a process by no means confined to the case of mental illness. The symbiotic relationship between psychiatry and insanity ... is merely a particularly important example ... of a much more general trend in the social control practices of modern societies. Elites in such societies over about the past century and a half have increasingly sought to rationalize and legitimize their control of all sorts of deviant and troublesome elements by consigning them to the ministrations of experts. No longer content to rely on vague cultural definitions of, and informal responses to, deviation, rational-bureaucratic western societies have increasingly delegated this task to groups of people who claim, or are assumed to have, special competence in these areas.[15]

In fact the use of the term 'delegation' in this quotation is questionable, as Scull clearly demonstrates that the emerging psychiatric profession actively sought to gain control of the mad business precisely at a time when it became clear that there were lucrative pickings to be had. Prior to 1750, the mentally disordered were generally not recognized as a separate category – they were heaped together with the poor and indigent and considered to be a family or communal responsibility. However, as the century progressed, new and more institutionalized methods of dealing with such groups were established in order to contain such problematical and potentially disruptive elements. Private madhouses were also founded as it became clear that the better classes were willing to pay handsomely in order to avoid the embarrassment of daily contact with mad relatives. Such madhouses were often run by laymen, but increasingly apothecaries, surgeons and physicians were attracted to the trade, particularly as they could claim that they had unique medical methods of achieving cures. As most methods of treatment were cure-alls which were quite indiscriminate in their application, it was a simple matter to include 'mental' illnesses alongside other forms of illness as legitimate targets for such treatment. Patients were therefore purged or bled or administered vomits or drugs with increasing enthusiasm.

However, as Scull is careful to point out, lay enthusiasm for such treatments proved more fickle. A number of reformers became increasingly concerned at the often cruel and inhumane régimes to which the insane were exposed. It was in this context that William Tuke developed an alternative approach at the York Retreat. Tuke's work (not mentioned by Wing in his account) was in part a reaction to the abuses that had been uncovered at the York Asylum but it is clear that his work achieved national importance, particularly through the publication in 1813 of his book, *A Description of the Retreat.*

Tuke was generally distrustful of doctors but allowed them to visit the Retreat. He concluded that they had little to offer his patients, although he did acknowledge that the warm baths they recommended did seem to help melancholics. Tuke's alternative approach viewed the insane as essentially child-like – they required humane treatment within a framework of re-education for life. Whenever possible, they were to be treated as rational and responsible. The Retreat was able to claim a high success rate with its patients, and these successes helped to fuel the rising tide of criticism of the existing asylums and madhouses. A series of Select Committees began investigations, and their reports revealed a catalogue of scandals and abuses (often involving ineffective or damaging medical treatments) and alarmingly high mortality rates.

As Scull clearly documents, these Select Committees were extremely critical both of medical forms of treatment and medical practitioners; physicians such as Best and Monro who were responsible for administering asylums were given a very rough ride when cross-examined by the Committees. More crucially, the Committees were hostile to the medical profession's claims to have special jurisdiction over the mentally ill. One lay witness to the Select Committee's deliberation had the following to say about whether medical men should be allowed to assume the roles of 'inspectors' or 'controllers' in relation to the mentally ill:

I think they are the most unfit of any class of persons. In the first place, *from every enquiry I have made, I am satisfied that medicine has little or no effect on the disease, and the only reason for their selection is the confidence which is placed in their being able to apply a remedy to the malady.* They are all persons interested more or less. It is extremly difficult in examining either the public Institutions or private houses not to have a strong impression upon your mind, that medical men derive a profit in some shape or form from those different establishments ... The rendering therefore, [of] any interested class of persons the Inspectors and Controllers, I hold to be mischievous in the greatest possible degree.[16]

Another even more hostile witness who had monitored the practices of one of the most famous medical 'specialists' in the field (Dr Best at the York Asylum) pointed out that the mortality rate at the asylum fell from twenty a year to only four following Dr Best's departure.

In practice, the majority of the members of the Committees accepted such views, since they recommended that asylums should be supervised by laymen and not doctors. The Bills of 1816–17 based on the deliberations of the Select Committees were passed by the House of Commons but were blocked by the House of Lords, largely because the Lords were opposed to reform in any shape or form. The medical profession therefore won a fragile victory over their opponents who viewed moral treatment as a more humane and effective approach.

However, as Scull points out, there were other reasons why the medical view gained ascendancy. Moral treatment, because of its non-technicality, did not encourage the emergence of an organized professional group which would seek to prevent other groups from adopting it. In addition, exponents of moral treatment proved largely incapable of confronting the medical profession both at a theoretical level and at a descriptive (linguistic) level. The language of madness remained that of medicine. These factors combined to make moral treatment vulnerable to a takeover bid from the medical profession – and this, as Scull carefully documents, is precisely what happened.

After the failure of a further Bill in 1819, there was a veritable spate of books on mental illness written by members of the medical profession. Scull insists that these did little more than to create an extensive body of largely spurious knowledge which served a useful purpose in mystifying and confusing lay opinion. In the same period medical degrees began to include the study of mental illness, so that medical men could substantiate their claims to have esoteric knowledge not possessed by lay competitors. More crucially, medical practitioners began to advance theories about mental illness which contained a significant ideological component of great value in confronting lay critics. Using Descartes' fundamental postulate that there was a split between mind and body, they insisted that the mind (an immortal, immaterial essence equivalent to the soul) was forced to operate in this world through the medium of the brain. However, the mind itself was, because of its very nature, incapable of being deranged or rendered imperfect. Only the brain can be damaged, so that a derangement in, for example, understanding, could no longer be considered as primarily a psychological phenomenon but as a direct manifestation of a disease process involving the centre in the nervous system upon which the exercise of understanding depended. This sophisticated, but clearly reductionist, model naturally carried with it the corollary that only the medical profession, with its expertise in treating bodily disease, could be legitimately involved in treating the mentally disordered. A further corollary must also be noted – it was argued that moral treatment, since it stressed the therapeutic value of a 'physical' form of treatment (the administration of hot baths), could only be legitimately supervised by doctors.

Many of these arguments have a remarkably contemporary ring about them, at least as far as our ears are concerned, but it is clear from Scull's work that they were the ideological smokescreen which the medical profession used to establish its dominance. The profession's first clear-cut victory came with the passing of the 1828 Act, which contained the stipulation that all asylums should have medical supervision. Initially this supervision was for physical complaints only, but once the door was open to the physicians they were able to undermine lay supervision and gain effective control of the running of the asylum. With the passing of the 1845 Lunatics Act, the medical profession's claims to have the sole right to treat the mentally disordered received statutory endorsement – doctors now controlled the only legitimate institutions for the treatment of the insane, and also began to profoundly influence the way that mental disorder was to be construed by lay opinion.

It is precisely in this period that the psychiatrists can be talked about collectively as belonging to a profession. In 1851 the Association of Medical Officers of Asylums and Hospitals for the Insane was founded and by 1853 it was publishing its own 'Asylum Journal'. Needless to say, the Journal propagated the view that insanity was purely a disease of the brain and that the physician was now the responsible guardian of the lunatic and must ever remain so. However, two major difficulties confronted the profession in this period. First, it was difficult in practice to demonstrate that organic pathology did in fact exist, and second, the profession's claims to produce effective cures were shown to be spurious. Interestingly, Scull cites Bucknill and Tuke's textbook published in 1858 as crucial evidence on this point. This textbook was recognized as the standard one, and yet it contained the following damaging admission: 'in the chronic stages of insanity active remedies are rarely admissible, except to obviate some intercurrent condition, which produces too much disturbance and danger to be permitted to run a natural course and wear itself out. In recent insanity with symptoms of physical disturbance of little violence and urgency, active medicinal treatment may often times be dispensed with.'

Admissions such as these, coupled with the fact that there were no universally agreed methods of treatment anyway, left asylum doctors in a highly vulnerable position. However, as Scull persuasively argues, they were able to maintain their position of dominance precisely because of their earlier victory over lay opposition. Scull makes his point with such telling clarity that we quote it in full:

By the Acts of 1828 and 1845, the medical profession had acquired a virtually exclusive right to direct the treatment of the insane. Thereafter, its concern became one of maintaining, rather than obtaining, a monopolistic position, a situation where those in possession generally operate from a tactically superior position. In this instance, the medical profession's control of asylums, the only legitimate institutions for the treatment of insanity, effectively shut out all potential competitors; for the latter would have had to oppose unsubstantiated claims to demonstrated performance. Furthermore, the asylum doctors' institutional base gave them a powerful leverage for getting the community to utilize their services (thereby indirectly supporting their professional authority), quite apart from whether those doing so were convinced of their competence. For while employment of the asylum by the relatives of 'crazy' people or by local Poor Law authorities did not necessarily reflect acceptance of the superintendent's claims or his esoteric definition of what was 'really' wrong with the troublesome people they sent him: yet still their ready use of his services unavoidably added to the aura of legitimacy surrounding his activities. So long as his services were in such demand, it was difficult to avoid concluding that he was performing a useful and valuable task for the community.

If the attractions of a convenient institution in which to dump the undesirable sufficed to ensure at least the passive acquiescence of the asylum doctors' true clients, the families and parish officials, in their continued existence, it should be quite clear that their nominal clients, the asylums' inmates, had little choice but to cooperate in sustaining their definition of the situation. Freidson has argued that, for the profession of medicine as a whole, a significant monopoly could not occur until a secure and practical technology of work was developed. In essence this was because doctors could not force clients to come to them, they had to *attract* them. Fortunately for psychiatrists, they formed an exception to this generalization, because of the peculiar structural characteristics of their practice. Once they had secured control over asylums, they no longer had to attract clients – the institution did that for them. And once patients were obtained, they formed literally a captive audience held in a context which gave immense power to their captors. Consequently, psychiatry was able, like the scholarly professions, to survive solely by gaining the interest and patronage of a special, powerful sponsor without having to gain general lay confidence.[17]

While agreeing with much of Scull's argument contained in this quotation, we would wish to modify Freidson's notion that a monopolistic position can be straightforwardly related to the development of 'a secure and practical technology of work'.[18] We have little space to explore this point here, but it is difficult to see how Freidson's position can be substantiated historically. The passing of the 1858 Medical Registration Act, which gave an effective monopoly to the medical profession in Britain, appears to pre-date any major discoveries which could provide medicine with a valid technology. We would therefore see the issue far more in ideological and class terms – it is perhaps churlish to criticize Scull on this ground, given the value of his work; but we do feel that he pays insufficient attention to the social and political context in which the psychiatric profession emerged.

In doing so, he follows closely in the footsteps of Freidson, whose contributions to understanding the nature of the medical profession have a strongly internalist bias, as Waitzkin and Waterman[19] have pointed out. We would therefore seek to add another dimension to Scull's argument: as Skultans[20] has pointed out in her commentary on ideas about insanity in the nineteenth century, the latter half of the century was a period of significant economic change – of a movement away from *laissez-faire* policies towards increasing state intervention as class divisions hardened. It is precisely in this period that 'psychiatric Darwinism' (to use Skultans' term) emerges with great force. Darwin's ideas, particularly as developed by Spencer and Galton, gave new force to the idea of incurability, since this could be attributed to hereditary causation.[21] Custodial care could therefore be justified as the only means of care possible. Asylums, therefore, became increasingly prison-like in their operation, but the medical profession was able to maintain its control of them largely because it could correctly insist that the inmates required extensive medical care on account of their poor physical condition.

But this is not to say that the asylum superintendents had absolute power. Legally speaking, they were merely salaried employees of the individual asylum committees, and at times these committees did use their powers to dismiss superintendents. According to Scull, the committees retained a profound scepticism about the value of medical superintendents, who were often seen as merely 'ornamental'. Asylum superintendents were also vulnerable in another respect: the actual contractual terms upon which they worked meant that they lived in almost total isolation (just like their patients). They were forced to live in asylum accommodation and to give up private practice. Their isolation is also reflected in the weak links between the asylum superintendents and the main section of the medical profession. Until very recently, psychiatry has been treated as a peripheral speciality of marginal importance to medicine, but it is important to stress that its segregation took a legal form until the passing of the 1959 Mental Health Act. The Act was significant in that it allowed mental patients to be treated within any type of hospital facility rather than in mental hospitals alone. As we have argued elsewhere,[22] the impetus to establish psychiatric units in general hospitals can be seen as the final attempt of the psychiatric profession to desegregate itself. Ironically, it appears that to be an asylum superintendent in the nineteenth century was to tar oneself with the brush that also tarred one's patients.

But it is essential to establish how the asylum superintendents were able to retain their monopoly in the face of the difficulties that confronted them. As the asylums became increasingly larger the superintendents retreated from personal contact with their charges, busying themselves with administrative duties. In practice, therefore, they became insulated from the reality of the asylums they controlled. They now actively sought administrative roles, since their role as architects of medical cures was clearly void. In the earliest asylums the medical profession had accumulated such administrative powers largely for reasons of economy – asylum committees were loath to pay an administrator and a physician when the latter could do both jobs. As the asylum grew in size it would have been a logical step to appoint a lay administrator to relieve the physician of administrative burdens but, as Scull demonstrates, such moves were (for obvious reasons) vehemently opposed by the physicians, who were able to convince the committees that asylums were in fact hospitals to be run exclusively by medical men.

So the solution to the problem of increasing size was solved by the appointment of assistant physicians (not lay administrators), ostensibly appointed to take care of the physical ailments of the patients. However, it is clear from Scull's careful documentation that they duly reflected the passion for pathological investigation which dominated medicine at that time. In 1870, 42 per cent of the patients who died in asylums were given an autopsy; by 1890, the figure had reached 76.6 per cent. The issue goes deeper than this – obviously the assistants, like the asylum superintendents, were keen to minimize the amount of contact that they had to have with their disturbed and disturbing patients. It was evidently both scientifically and socially more respectable to work with corpses than patients: the day-to-day tasks of handling the patients were, in fact, left to asylum attendants, recruited, according to contemporary accounts, from the very same strata that provided the asylums with the majority of their clientele.

In the final analysis, Scull attributes the victory of the asylum superintendents in retaining control of the asylums to two factors – the cult of science and public indifference:

I suggest that such a persistent, almost wilful blindness [to the failure of medical treatments] derives from something more than the sacred and hence unquestioned quality with which modern societies have endowed science and certified expertise. It is true, of course, that such unexamined deference is habitually exhibited in its most acute form in the realm of medicine. Indeed, the doctor–patient relationship is so structured as to demand routinely that the client abdicate his own reasoning capacity. In its place is fostered a naïve child-like faith that the physician is operating in the patient's best interests; and that, while he does so, he is guided by an esoteric training and knowledge giving him insights which are beyond the powers of ordinary mortals to grasp or understand. But, when all is said and done, modern medicine, much of the time at least, has results, if not God, on its side. English psychiatry at the end of the nineteenth century (and most of the 'experts' currently engaged in the control of deviance) clearly did (do) not.

And yet, if asylums, and the activities of those running them, did not transform their inmates into upright citizens, they did at least get rid of troublesome people for the rest of us. By not inquiring too deeply into what went on behind asylum walls, and by not being too sceptical of the officially constructed reality, people were (are) rewarded with a comforting reassurance about the essentially benign character of their society and the way it dealt (deals) with its deviants and misfits. Granting a few individuals the status and perquisites ordinarily thought to be reserved for those with genuine expertise and esoteric knowledge was a small price to pay for the satisfaction of knowing that crazy people were getting the best treatment science could provide, and for the comfortable feelings which could be aroused by contemplating the contrast between the present 'humane' and 'civilized' approach to the 'mentally ill' with the barbarism of the past.[23]

We have quoted this passage at length because it raises many themes which we wish to explore as we extend our argument to include twentieth-century developments in psychiatry; but at this point it is necessary for us to draw heavily on some recent work by David Ewins which is complementary to Scull's, although it explores the period between 1890 and 1960.[24]

Ewins shares Scull's view that the medical profession's role in relation to the mentally disordered was paradoxical – by the end of the century it had consolidated its claim to be solely responsible for treating insanity, but it could only carry out this function within the constraints of a complex administrative and legal framework. The latter had been greatly modified by the 1890 Lunacy Act, which established a series of complex safeguards against wrongful detention on the grounds of insanity. Ewins is particularly interested in the legal changes which occurred firstly with the passing of the Mental Treatment Act of 1930, and then the far more 'radical' Mental Health Act of 1959.

The explanation for these changes is to be found partly in the changing social and political conditions of this period, and partly in developments within medicine itself. Ewins argues that the success of medicine in devising new and effective methods of treating syphilitic patients in the period leading up to the First World War created a climate of opinion that once again facilitated the acceptance of the medical view of insanity as 'illness'. This in turn strengthened the medical profession's claim to ultimate control over the detention and treatment of the mentally ill without the restrictions of detailed legal regulations and safeguards.

But the success of the new methods would not of itself have been decisive in determining the ascendancy of the medical profession. Indeed, one has to question whether the new methods devised in this period *were* generally successful. Ewins himself does not argue this point in sufficient detail, but we feel it is more convincing to postulate that the important point about the new methods of treatment was not that they were demonstrably successful but that they were construed as being successful.

For that the final quarter of the nineteenth century was a crucial turning point in the history of medicine, and the changes that occurred in this period profoundly influenced psychiatry. As George Rosen has demonstrated, theories about the nature and causation of physical illness underwent considerable changes as a result of the epoch-making discoveries of bacteriologists like Koch and Pasteur. Their success in understanding and eventually treating infectious diseases resulted in the establishment of a paradigm within medicine which stressed the importance of pathological processes within the individual, while largely ignoring the social and economic factors that inevitably influenced disease processes. We need to digest this rather obvious point in greater detail because it has crucial implications for the history of psychiatry.

Rosen's approach is particularly important since he has explored the impact of social and political changes on the development of both medicine and the profession of medicine, not just in this period but also throughout the nineteenth century. Significantly, he has paid close attention to the impact of the French Revolution on the development of the medical profession on the Continent. In his own words he sees the Revolution as implanting 'ideas of public interest and social utility which provided the seed in which germinated views of the relation among health, medicine and society. The men of 1789 and 1793 could not foresee the consequences of their thoughts and acts. The triumph of the machine and the concentration of capital were still in the future, but it was in terms of the situation created by these developments that the men of 1848 endeavoured to apply the ideas of their predecessors. *Social* medicine, the idea of 1848, must be seen as the fruit of this historical process.'[25]

Rosen argues that the rapid industrialization and urbanization that occurred in France between 1830 and 1870 imposed a series of economic and social stresses that influenced very profoundly the evolution of French thought and action. During this period an energetic group of physicians and hygienists had been carrying out surveys and statistical studies of living conditions among workers in urban communities. Practical experience acquired during the Revolutionary and Napoleonic wars had made many French physicians alert to health problems. At the same time, political and social theorists, such as Fourier, Saint-Simon, Comte, Proudhon and many others, influenced French medicine, so that certain sections of it were fermented with a spirit of social change. Many doctors were in direct contact with the social realities of industrialization and the profound effects it had on the lives of the working class.

In 1838 Rochoux coined the term 'social hygiene' to describe a category of social policy that would be concerned with establishing a legal and administrative framework for providing minimum health standards. Ten years later, at the height of the 1848 Revolution, Guérin appealed to the French medical profession to contribute to the good of society. Guérin divided his social medicine into four parts: social physiology, social pathology, social hygiene and social therapy. These were to deal, respectively, with the relation between the physical and mental condition of a population and its laws or other institutions; the study of social problems in relation to health and disease; measures for health promotion and disease prevention; and the provision of medical and other conditions that societies may experience.

Guérin's idea of social medicine obviously awarded the medical profession a key role in running society. Throughout Europe, the profession was struggling to establish itself as a unified entity (with uniform training and uniform payment for the services it rendered), which would be able to provide more and better care for the majority of the population. Not surprisingly, the first proposals for a national medical service also began to emerge in this period. But what became of this movement within medicine? In France, the period of political reaction following the failure of the 1848 Revolution put paid to such proposals. Some German physicians, such as Neumann, Virchow and Leubuscher, were profoundly influenced by the theories of social medicine in France. In 1847, Neumann had issued a manifesto arguing that 'medical science is intrinsically and essentially a social science, and as long as this is not recognized in practice we shall have to be satisfied with an empty shell and a sham'. Virchow formulated the idea somewhat differently, stating that 'medicine is a social science and politics nothing but medicine on a grand scale'. But, as Rosen points out, the proponents of such ideas were not dreaming of some utopian situation: they utilized their approach to formulate definite principles from which a programme of action could be derived. The exact details of such programmes are not our concern here, but it is obvious that such physicians saw the task of medicine in a much broader light than their biologically- and pathologically-orientated colleagues.

The attempt of these men to turn medicine in a sociological and preventive direction was abortive, since the failure of the revolution in Germany created a political climate hostile to social medicine. At the same time, developments in other scientific disciplines (especially biology and physics) began to influence the development of medicine. As Rosen comments:

The natural sciences developed rapidly and achieved enormous prestige in medicine, and the emergence of medical bacteriology seemed to answer the problem of disease causation. Under these conditions it was not difficult to overlook the significance of the relationship between the patient and his environment.[26]

Or, as a leading German bacteriologist, Emil Behring, declared in 1894, the study of infectious diseases could now be pursued unswervingly without being side-tracked by social considerations and reflections on social policy.

Rosen's discussion of the developments within medicine concentrates mainly on France and Germany, but he does point out that there were some developments towards an idea of social medicine in Britain, although these were a pale imitation of the developments on the Continent. Continental and British medicine became more unified in their development precisely because of the successes of medical bacteriology. However – and this is the crux of the point we are trying to make – as medicine became more scientific, more concerned with measurement and classification and the theory of pathological processes, it became less humanistic and tended to treat the patient as an object. In *Medical Nemesis*[27] Illich has graphically argued this point: '... as the doctor's interest shifted from the sick to sickness, the hospital became a museum of sickness. The wards were full of indigent people who offered their bodies as spectacles to any physician willing to treat them.'

In the same period, a basic shift occurred in the taking of medical case histories.[28] In the Hippocratic tradition, a clinical history was a history of a human being who suffered and who had symptoms. In the second half of the nineteenth century, however, as pathology developed as a science, doctors became more and more preoccupied with establishing the history of a particular disease process (*historia morbi*). The individual, his social relations and his problems of living then faded into insignificance as attention was focused upon the symptoms and their bodily manifestations. Illich has argued that this process became all the more powerful and irresistible as the medical profession was able to develop effective cures for a wide range of diseases. As a result of this very real power, the profession increasingly gained control over defining what is illness and what is health.

This process also occurred in relation to mental illness. The discoveries associated with the successful treatment of general paresis of the insane (culminating in Wagner Jauregg's malarial treatment, for which he was awarded a Nobel Prize) was construed as undeniable evidence that all mental disorders were illnesses. Thus, psychiatry was able to capitalize both on its limited success with GPI and on the general advances being made in medicine. With hindsight, we now can establish just how limited these successes were: McKeown, Cochrane, Powles and many other writers have demonstrated that major changes in living standards and life-style have contributed far more to changes in health than innovations in therapy, and even Wing concedes that 'the more dramatic advances in diagnosis and in the treatment of those diseases that affect individuals (as opposed to large groups) have probably contributed significantly only since the second quarter of the present century'.[29]

Clearly it was not due to the limited successes of psychiatry that the medical profession was able to dominate the deliberations of the Royal Commission on Lunacy (1924–7). To explain this domination, we must accept Scull's points concerning the monopoly position gained by the profession and also argue that the other main reason for its domination was an ideological one.

The latter point has been argued in some detail by Ewins. He insists that the categorization of forms of deviant behaviours as mental illness is an especially advantageous form of social control. Any threat or potential threat to the existing political and social conditions of society can be eliminated or greatly lessened by forcing the deviant to enter the sick role. His actions can then be invalidated, since they are seen either as meaningless or as mere symptoms whose meaning is to be deciphered by the psychiatrist. The deviant is no longer held responsible for his own behaviour – his illness is simply something that happens to him, over which he has no control. He is thus entirely in the control of the doctor, who alone has the power to cure him.

Ewins argues that the power of medical explanations of deviant behaviour lies precisely in their ability to divest such behaviour of any political significance. If deviant behaviours are construed as pathological symptoms resulting from a disease process, there is no longer any question of conceptualizing them in other ways. (For example, there would be no question of examining the content of the symptoms to see whether they reflect the effects of having to cope with the alienating effects of living in a capitalist form of society.)

But Ewins is also concerned to explore other features of medicalization. In this connection he draws on the work of Parsons,[30] who points out that criminals, since they are labelled and extruded from the company of upright citizens, must be prevented by coercion from joining up with their fellow criminals. There is no such problem, however, when the form of deviance is illness rather than criminality. A sick person's status is conditionally legitimated when he willingly makes himself dependent upon other people who are not sick – friends, family members, doctors, etc. – rather than on fellow sufferers. This creates real barriers to group formation among the sick, and little possibility of positive legitimation. The sick role thus not only isolates and insulates the sick person, but also exposes him to very powerful forces compelling him to become reintegrated into society as a fully participating member.

In Parsons' system, these processes are seen as natural and non-problematic: entry into the sick role is merely one of several routes that individuals may take in response to personal crises. But, as Waitzkin and Waterman[31] have pointed out, the sick role can be viewed as a particularly effective mechanism of social control, since it permits limited deviance to occur, but at the same time protects the stability of the social system. It is for this reason that Ewins insists that the medicalization of mental disorder has to be understood against the background of an emerging political consensus which maintained that problems of health, and particularly mental illness, were not a matter for party politics. He correctly stresses that the Labour Party played a crucial role in contributing and shaping this consensus, but he fails to develop a sufficiently detailed discussion of the relationship between developments in capitalism and the development of the Labour Party as a vehicle for reformist politics.

At this point, therefore, we shall diverge once more from Ewin's account, turning instead to an analysis put forward by Bernard Semmel[32] in his book *Imperialism and Social Reform*. Semmel is concerned primarily with exploring the relationship between the development of imperialism and changes in welfare policies between 1890 and the First World War. In his analysis of the economic bases of social reform, he does not specifically discuss services for the mentally disordered, but his general analysis clearly provides a deeper understanding of the reasons for the changes that occurred here in embryonic form in the 1920s and 1930s and more strikingly after the Second World War. However, in order to introduce this analysis, it is necessary to make some general comments about Semmel's approach.

Semmel views the provision of social and welfare reforms within a specific historical context – one in which the ruling class in Britain was faced with containing an increasingly sophisticated and politically conscious working class. Many politicians saw Bismarck's Germany as the most suitable model to be emulated, since the 'state socialism' he had introduced in the 1880s had been consciously designed to stem social and political discontent in the working class and to undermine the growing strength of the German socialist movement. An alternative solution to the problem was suggested by Cecil Rhodes, who argued that in order to avoid class conflicts at home it was necessary to develop a policy of imperialist domination. As he graphically put it, 'The Empire . . . is a bread and butter question. If you want to avoid civil war you must become imperialists.'[33]

British politics in the period prior to the First World War were dominated by such discussions. The majority of both Liberal and Tory politicians accepted that imperialism was essential in order to provide the economic basis for social reform in Britain; moreover, the influential Fabian Society had also developed a policy of advocating imperialist policies. They therefore decided to support what Semmel calls the liberal-imperialist wing of the Liberal Party led by Earl Rosebery, whose view of the relationship between imperialism and social reform is summarized by the following quotations cited by Semmel:

An Empire . . . requires as its first condition an imperial race – a race vigorous and industrious and intrepid . . . where you promote health and arrest disease, where you convert an unhealthy citizen into a healthy one, where you exercise your authority to promote sanitary conditions . . . you in doing your duty are also working for the Empire.

Issues such as educational, housing and temperance reform were linked by Rosebery to the idea of efficiency:

a condition of national fitness equal to the demands of our Empire – administrative, parliamentary, commercial, educational, physical, moral, naval and military fitness – so that we should make the best of our admirable raw material.

Since the Fabians believed that they could achieve their goals of social reform by converting the leaders of the existing parties (a policy of 'permeation'), they were naturally attracted to Rosebery's view. In keeping with these political moves, the Fabian Society therefore preferred to drop references to socialism, since this term inevitably carried with it overtones of class-oriented politics. The term 'collectivist' was used instead to describe their policies, which were primarily concerned with the promotion of the national interest. The latter could be most efficiently achieved by ensuring that the imperial economy (organized on a collectivist basis) was directed by an élite of experts. The efficiency of the economy would be the basis for improving the conditions of the most depressed classes of the community.

The Fabians' corporatist ideas clearly influenced many groups within the Labour Party, but Semmel demonstrates convincingly that there was also a crucial ideological link between the Fabians and the various political movements in which Sir Oswald Mosley played a part. His rapid political evolution was entirely consistent. From being a Tory he became first an 'Independent', then a member of the Labour Party (eventually with a Cabinet post), and finally the leader of the British Union of Fascists. His corporatist doctrines were often indistinguishable from policies put forward by the Fabians, whose basic authoritarianism is particularly clearly illustrated in relation to their social welfare policies.

These policies have particular relevance to our arguments concerning the provision of new forms of services for the mentally disordered. For example, the Minority Report of the 1909 Royal Commission on the Poor Laws (written by Sidney and Beatrice Webb) contained some remarkably authoritarian recommendations. It suggested that vigorous campaigns to improve the health of the poor should be undertaken, irrespective of the consent of the people involved. These suggestions foreshadowed the powers given to doctors under the Mental Health Act in 1959, but other sections of the recommendations are also significant since they argue in favour of positive welfare legislation and attack notions of *laissez-faire*.

The Fabians and the policy-makers of the Labour Party played an important part in this process, but they were not, of course, solely responsible for formulating welfare policies. The reforms introduced by the Liberal Government from 1908 onwards (concerned with working conditions, housing, health insurance and old age pensioners) were formulated by the left-wingers in the party, who were not necessarily influenced by the Fabians, although ironically their policies were indistinguishable from those of the Fabians. Most sections of the Conservative Party bitterly opposed such policies, but the growing power of the Labour Party, reflecting basic developments in the working class, forced the Conservatives to accept and even endorse many of the policies introduced originally by the Liberal Party and later by the Labour Party as it inherited the mantle of the Liberals. This consensus between the Conservative and Labour parties emerged most clearly during and after the Second World War. The Beveridge programme for post-war reconstruction, which included proposals for a national health service, had been drawn up during a period of coalition, but the heavy defeat that the Conservatives received at the hands of the Labour Party in 1945 made it clear to them that they had to accept the basic tenets of the so-called 'welfare state'.

The changes embodied in the 1930 Mental Treatment Act, and more crucially in the 1959 Mental Health Act, must therefore be seen as an example of the growing consensus over health and welfare issues. Both major parties were concerned with preserving the existing political and economic system, and were thus united in seeking to eliminate or control any social phenomenon that challenged the *status quo*. Both parties were also wedded to policies designed to ameliorate social conditions, and both placed great stress on productivity and economic growth. Since 'unproductiveness' was now viewed in much the same spirit as pauperism, new forms of medical treatment (notably drug therapy) which enabled the mentally ill to be returned to productive work were looked upon with great interest.

But, as Ewins points out, these new forms of treatment had wider implications: while development of community care was linked closely to its success in preventing prolonged hospitalization, it also involved more effective methods of social control. Psychiatric medicine could now not only return patients to productiveness, but could also re-socialize them in step with the norms and values of society.

These developments were particularly appropriate from the reformist point of view of the Labour Party. Psychiatrists could now be viewed as performing a similar function to that of social workers. Part of this function would necessarily involve re-socializing deviant members of society so that they would accept the 'objective reality' dictated by the more powerful groups in society. This essentially authoritarian aspect of reformist thinking also stresses the importance of 'experts' in deciding how people should regulate their lives. It is therefore not surprising that the Minority Report on the Poor Law also emphasized the importance of doctors in regulating the lives of the poor. Clearly, psychiatrists can execute such a function in very powerful ways, and in this context Ewins draws particular attention to the use of mental welfare agencies as last resorts for younger, 'difficult' members of society who have been through the hands of the educational and possibly also of the legal authorities. He also insists that almost all contemporary psychiatric practice operates in a similar way.

The recent extension of psychiatry to include community care is therefore of fundamental importance. Indeed, Ewins concludes:

;;. as a result of the introduction of community care ... psychiatrists and mental welfare agencies could be increasingly integrated into the elaborate social welfare fabric (constructed largely by the Labour Party with the increasing acquiescence and support of the Conservative Party) behind which lay the belief that social problems could be eradicated by positive efforts to ameliorate social conditions.[34]

Labour Party policy-makers reciprocated by emphasizing the necessity of moving towards community care but at the same time, given their deference to expert opinion and their desire not to antagonize the medical profession, accepted the diverse nature of mental illness. Both sides benefited from this exchange – the medical profession gained prestige and power, while the Labour Party was able effectively to remove discussions of mental illness from the political arena, since mental illness merely became a 'social problem' which could be ameliorated; no longer was it construed as an endemic feature of a class society, which only a socialist reconstruction of society could attempt to eradicate in any fundamental way.

Ewin's argument appears to be rather programmatic (particularly as we have presented it here, owing to limitations on space), but it is well supported by the analysis he makes of the political background of the Mental Treatment Act and the Mental Health Act. He clearly demonstrates the Labour Government's role in ensuring that there was a radical break with the principles underlying the 1890 Lunacy Act, which had been preoccupied with defending the rights of the individual against unlawful committal to a mental asylum. For example, the Royal Commission on Lunacy and Mental Disorder (1924–7) had stressed the need to move towards a medical view of mental illness but had recommended the retention of the judicial authority in all cases of the detention of the mentally ill. The Labour Government, however, insisted on including a provision whereby 'non-volitional' patients (i.e. those judged to be incapable of expressing willingness to enter a mental hospital) could be detained on medical authority alone for a period of six months or a year. As the

Minister of Health of the time insisted, this provision was 'the heart of the Bill'. But it represented the first crucial move towards removing legal constraints on the activities of the medical profession with regard to detaining the mentally ill.

This provision was also important to Labour Party policy-makers since it enshrined a crucial element of their reformist thinking. The Government therefore not only ensured that any amendment that threatened the central provision of the Bill was defeated, but also effectively curtailed detailed discussion of many of its provisions by using the technique of closure motions. The Labour Government thus achieved its aim of granting increased power to the medical profession. However, the 1930 Act was clearly transitional – as Ewins remarks:

. . . at the medical level . . . there was still a marked tendency to regard many 'lunatics' as incurable and suitable only for detention . . . at the political level there was still substantial opposition to this movement away from the legalistic approach to the detention of the mentally ill.

By 1959, changes in therapy combined with changes in political attitudes to remove the obstacles to the general acceptance of the medical view of mental illness. The establishment of the National Health Service in 1949 contributed to these developments since it resulted in the first steps towards the integration of the mental health services with the general health services – a process that tended to reinforce the acceptance of the medical view of mental illness.

The Mental Health Act of 1959, like the Mental Treatment Act of 1930, was preceded by a Royal Commission; but whereas the previous Commission had been composed mostly of lawyers with only two medical representatives, the 1957 Commission was dominated by the medical profession. Irrespective of their political and professional background, both Commissions accepted the medical view of mental disorder, though they differed significantly in their actual functioning. The Report of the 1957 Commission shows that opposition to granting the medical profession increased powers was far more muted – only five organizations submitting evidence supported the retention of judicial powers.

Ewins also analyses the contribution made by the legal profession to the findings of the two Royal Commissions. The profession, as a whole, did not feel its interests threatened by a movement towards medical rather than judicial control of the mentally disordered, because of fundamental social and political changes. He argues that while the legal profession evinced great concern for the liberty of the subject with regard to the compulsory commitment of the insane in a period dominated by the ethics of individualism and laissez-faire ... it would not oppose the movement towards extending the powers of compulsory commitment in an era of increasing state intervention and social welfare, particularly since such opposition would become increasingly futile and inimical to the interests of the profession, as consensus between the political parties with regard to social welfare (including treatment of the mentally ill) became established.[35]

The legal members of both Commissions therefore typically accepted the medical view of mental disorder and accepted that members of the medical profession should play the key role in committal procedures. But the most clear-cut indication of the acceptance of the medical view is the lack of opposition to the recommendations of the 1957 Commission, which removed the necessity for the automatic review of the grounds upon which patients were detained in hospitals. Automatic review was replaced by the proposal that patients should only have a right of appeal to a tribunal, since it was argued that a formal procedure might harm the welfare of a patient. The same argument was used to justify two further recommendations of the Commission concerning the functions of the tribunals. These were concerned with whether continued detention was necessary – not whether the original period of detention was justified or not. They were also to be given discretionary powers, which meant that they could decide whether proceedings were to be publicly reported, whether medical reports would be made available to the patient, or whether the reasons for particular decisions would be made available to patients and their relatives.

The 1957 Royal Commission Report (and the 1959 Mental Health Act which translated its recommendations into law) therefore represents the final victory of the medical profession in securing its claims to prime responsibility for the mentally disordered.

Our argument explaining why this victory was so long in being achieved has been long and somewhat tortuous, so it is worthwhile making one or two points by way of summary before once more commenting on the contemporary scene in Britain. The essence of Scull's argument is that the medical profession won control of the mad business for reasons that related to the needs of the profession, not the patients they sought to treat. As Ewins argues, the profession's final success was related to the economic and political changes that occurred as the Labour Party was emerging as a major political force. Psychiatry's claim to legitimacy has always been related to its pedigree as an offshoot of 'scientific medicine' – however, the conceptualization of medicine as 'science' is also highly problematic, being politically and historically determined.

At this point, the 'efficacy' issue also enters the argument. Most spokesmen for psychiatry will insist that it is entirely just that psychiatrists should have a unique and special role in terms of their relationship with their patients (and hence in terms of the law) because it is only psychiatrists who can administer the forms of treatment which are 'effective'. Of course, the issue of the nature of the 'effectiveness' is never really debated (and we have no space to enter into it here), but our reading of the history of psychiatry leads us to the conclusion that major changes both in health policies and in legal states of patients always takes place in a context in which the actual efficacy of the therapeutic methods of psychiatry has never been seriously explored. This will no doubt sound like heresy to many readers, but elsewhere we have reviewed evidence demonstrating that the policy of establishing psychiatric work in general hospitals did not stem from any major research programme.[36] Equally, both we and Scull,[37] in an entirely independent piece of researching, have attempted to demonstrate that the so-called 'drug revolution' involving the new psychotropic drugs introduced from 1954/5 onwards is highly questionable. The claims of this 'revolution' need to be confronted on a very broad basis, but a critical reading of the literature on the 'revolution' reveals some singularly contradictory findings. For example, Wing and Brown's meticulous study [38] of the chronic wards of three different hospitals showed that drug treatments were of no significance in contributing to the quality of life of the patients on these wards.

With the benefit of hindsight, it is possible to examine with more critical eyes the euphoria created by this so-called 'drug revolution' which was associated from 1954 onwards with a steady fall in the number of psychiatric beds occupied by patients. Clearly psychotropic drugs are 'effective' in relieving and controlling symptoms, but this does not mean that they develop a patient's ability to deal with his or her problems in any fundamental sense. In addition there is, of course, no logical reason why psychiatry's claim to be effective needs to impinge on the basic human rights of patients. After nearly twenty years' experience of the Mental Health Act, there is now both increasing concern about the way that the psychiatric profession has been a party to undermining the rights of patients[39] and increasing lay scepticism about the claims of the profession to really provide effective help.[40]

The way we have presented these issues here is very programmatic, and further research work is obviously required, but nevertheless in order to conclude our main argument we shall now raise some further issues concerning the implications of psychiatry's final victory. This victory occurred in a period when the state increasingly intervened to regulate and control more and more aspects of everyday living. The extension of the sick role, to encompass many forms of deviancy which reflect the basic conflicts in a class society more clearly and openly than issues relating to general health or illness, has obvious advantages to the ruling groups within that society. The psychiatric profession, operating from the standpoint of self-interest, has been a willing tool in this process of mystification, but there is a very real sense in which the profession creates and perpetuates the very problems which it claims to be able to solve. Ivan Illich[41] has been primarily responsible for drawing attention to such issues in relation to general medicine, but it is worthwhile spelling out some of the subtleties of the relationship between the psychiatrist and his clientele. There is a real sense in which the sick role can be exploited by the individual who enters it. The role absolves the patient from responsibility for his 'illness', and hence carries with it the implication that the patient is no longer the agency determining the therapeutic changes that occur. It is the doctor who performs this function, and in doing so he tends to engineer passivity in his patients. Passivity can, of course, cause immense difficulties when entrance to the sick role is the result of physical illness, but when entry occurs as a result of mental disorder the situation becomes much more problematic.

The process of becoming mentally ill involves crucial personal and interpersonal conflicts and adjustments which are clearly of a different order from those involved when the diagnosis is of physical disorder. Peter Sedgwick has, of course, argued a diametrically opposed view,[42] but in our opinion his analysis is largely spurious since it fails to take account of the meaning of illness for individuals who become 'ill' either physically or mentally. Admittedly the terms 'physically' or 'mentally' are arbitrary societally-derived labels, but to fail to see that they profoundly influence both the subsequent career of the individual and the way that he or she conceptualizes the problem is peculiarly myopic. (We have no space to explore this issue here although David

Morgan's article 'Explaining mental illness'[43] does much to clarify the many vexing theoretical issues in this area.)

Fortunately some recent work by the psychiatrist, R. D. Scott, has also provided many crucial insights into the processes of becoming mentally ill.[44] The process whereby an individual becomes 'mentally ill' typically begins within family settings which are, of course, particularly difficult to study.[45] By studying the families of his own patients, Scott has provided us with a rather different perspective from that offered by sociologists, such as Scheff. His studies have demonstrated that many patients are able to use their 'madness' not only to control and influence their close relatives but also to manipulate the psychiatrists, social workers and other professionals they encounter. Scott's work, therefore, provides a rather different picture of the psychiatrist/patient relationship. The psychiatrist certainly has great power in this relationship – powers of detention, powers of providing compulsory treatment, etc. – but the patient is often in a position to exploit the situation to his own advantage. Moreover, this ability to exploit some features of the sick role can turn into an inability ever to leave the role. The patient becomes trapped in the role and uses his manipulative skills to maintain the *status quo*. Any new therapeutic initiative taken by the psychiatrist or other member of staff is dislocated and eventually negated because neither the patient nor his family can tolerate any fundamental change.

Scott has coined the useful term 'treatment barrier' to describe the obstacles to effective therapy which are created by the culturally prescribed view of mental illness prevailing in Western society.[46] A central feature of this view is that the mentally disordered are ill and hence lack responsibility for their actions. Through his painstaking research work, and through his crisis intervention methods which flow from his research, Scott has attempted to confront these obstacles directly. In doing so, he has begun to open up many exciting new avenues for a contractually based therapy which avoids the social control dimension implicit in traditional psychiatric therapies. But, nevertheless, we cannot help pointing out the historically derived paradox in his work – Scott has made a significant contribution to confronting the medical model, but he has done so from the most unlikely base – namely Napsbury Hospital, a typical example of the kind of mental hospital to be found on the outskirts of any large city – which still reminds us that the medical model still dominates British psychiatry a hundred years on. Ironically, Scott has recently moved from

Napsbury to a psychiatric unit in a general hospital. Such units are, as we have argued elsewhere,[47] an even clearer reflection of the domination of the medical model within the mental health services. And yet it is from such a base that Scott will be continuing to operate his crisis intervention approach which is, of course, aimed primarily at preventing people in crises from entering the sick role as an opportunist solution to problems which are usually embedded in their interpersonal relationships.

Scott's work has been little recognized or valued within the psychiatric profession as a whole, but this is not surprising given the reactionary nature of the profession which we have documented in this chapter. So, in order to end our contribution in a way which validly reflects this history, it is necessary to turn away from Scott's innovations and consider the future of the profession as it is articulated by its main spokesmen. We have space for only one of these – no less a personage than Sir Keith Joseph who, in introducing the 1971 White Paper 'Hospital Services for the Mentally Ill', made the following observations:

Psychiatry is to join the rest of medicine . . . since the treatment of psychosis, neurosis and schizophrenia have been entirely changed by the drug revolution. People go into hospital with mental disorders and they are cured, and that is why we want to bring this branch of medicine into the scope of the 230 district general hospitals that are planned for England and Wales.[48]

Given the history of psychiatry which we have outlined in this chapter, need we say more?

5 French Anti-psychiatry

Sherry Turkle

Introduction

Three features make French anti-psychiatry very different from its Anglo-Saxon counterpart: its links with psychoanalysis, its links with Marxism and its grass roots base. This chapter introduces the French anti-psychiatric movement, using the contrast between French and Anglo-Saxon anti-psychiatry to bring the cultural specificity of the French movement into sharper focus. Thus, we stress French anti-psychiatry's relationship to French psychoanalysis, to other currents in French radical politics and to the student revolt of May–June 1968 whose aftermath seems to have conditioned a milieu receptive to anti-psychiatric ideas, particularly on the French Left.

In Freud's work are formulations of psychoanalysis as a radical doctrine with an implicit critique of social repression. In America, medical professionalization contributed to defusing much of what was most radical in his vision. The wedding of American psychoanalysis and psychiatry began as a marriage of convenience. When Freud's ideas appeared on the scene, American psychiatrists were in need of a new paradigm, and the first psychoanalysts wanted to use a medical affiliation to increase the legitimacy of the new doctrine. American psychoanalysis may well have paid a price for such expediencies. Torn from its base in the cultural sciences by an early (1927) decision by the American Psychoanalytic Association to limit the practice of psychoanalysis to medical doctors, American psychoanalysis became a psychiatric, medical and even corporate 'insider'. In its theoretical development it favored a psychoanalytic ego psychology where the predominant model is of a therapeutic alliance between the egos of analyst and patient in the service of a better adaptation to reality. American psychoanalysis was socialized or, perhaps, domesticated by American institutions and values. Although some analysts did use psychoanalytic insights as part of a critique of American life, they were exceptions to the general trend. In America, psychoanalysis did not develop a cutting edge as a language for social criticism. Thus, it is not surprising that *in the United States, anti-psychiatric stances have tended to imply anti-psychoanalytic ones.*

The development of psychoanalysis in France placed it in a radically different relationship to medicine and psychiatry. Far from being a psychiatric 'insider', it was a neglected, even stigmatized outsider. French psychiatry was strong and confident, wedded to a well-entrenched system of asylums on the one hand and to a neurological paradigm which had firm institutional bases in the hospital and university on the other.[1] The initial interest in psychoanalysis in France was strongest in the artistic community, particularly among the surrealists. Psychoanalysis remained an insignificant force in established French medicine and psychiatry until the mid-1960s. The marginality of psychoanalysis to psychiatry meant that *the critique of psychiatry which began to emerge in France after World War II did not develop against psychoanalysis but developed in close alliance with it.*

Tens of thousands of French mental patients had been allowed to starve to death during World War II; after the war the public horror at the atrocity gave momentum to a nascent movement for the reform of the psychiatric hospital system which had been growing up around the practice of psychiatrist François Tosquelles at Saint-Alban hospital. The principles behind the movement seem uncontroversial by today's standards, but they were radical in their challenge to the French asylum system as it stood in 1940. These principles included improvement of material conditions within the hospital, diminishing the then total separation between the hospital and the outside world, employing a therapeutic team whose members would engage patients in a variety of relationships and activities. The original group of reformers with Tosquelles (among them L. Bonnafe, G. Daumezon and L. Le Guillant) worked in an eclectic spirit of medical empiricism. Their goal was to rationalize and humanize an absurd and inhuman system and they were open to whatever they thought might help: drug therapy, group techniques, occupational therapy and certain psychoanalytic techniques. The reformers knew their success depended on major shifts in French social policy towards the mentally ill, and in particular on an end to the total social segregation of mental patients. Although the movement began with enthusiasm, the necessary changes in social policy did not materialize. When gestures came (such as a 1960 administrative circular which theoretically set up a French community mental health program – known in France as the *sectorisation*) they were unsupported by the funds needed to sustain them.

Today, the original reform movement has its spiritual descendants in attempts to rationalize French psychiatry. The group of contemporary reformers include the psychoanalysts who promoted a community health program as a pilot study in Paris' 13th *arrondissement.* This pilot, known as the *sectorisation*, became the model for a new national health policy after the May–June 1968 events: all of France is now broken up into community mental health 'sectors'. The analysts who set up the pilot sector were all committed anti-Lacanians and members of the Société Psychanalytique de Paris, the Paris Psychoanalytic Society, the oldest and most medically dominated of the four French psychoanalytic societies. In general, they see psychoanalysis as the technique which makes it possible for the psychiatric system to become an adequate solution to the medical and social problem of psychosis. For them, the major obstacle to psychiatric therapy is the hospital model of practice and they propose a marriage of psychiatric and flexible psychoanalytic ideas which will bring a modernized, supple psychiatry out into the community.[2]

According to this model, psychoanalysis exists to help psychiatry do its task better. The medical and psychiatric system and its hierarchies are accepted, not challenged. In the 13th *arrondissement*'s community mental health center, psychoanalytic power tends to reinforce medical authority: the entire institution operates by a kind of consensus about psychoanalysis, but for the non-physicians, access to psychoanalysis is through an identification with the psychiatrist-analyst-leader.

Before 1968 these reformers stood almost alone as representing French 'anti-psychiatry'. Today, their approach (which does not challenge the notion of cure, the role of psychiatry in masking social problems or the potential dangers of the sector) defines the position *against* which contemporary anti-psychiatric thought and action are developing. Current efforts in radical anti-psychiatry tend to be pro-Lacan and highly politicized.

Whereas American revisionists of Freud had strained to produce more 'optimistic' versions of his work which promised self improvement without calling society into question, in France, a post-1968 outpouring of interest in psychoanalysis began with interest in the work of Herbert Marcuse and Wilhelm Reich, two theorists whose effort is to make the links between psyche and society more explicit. Unlike its American counterpart, major currents in French psychoanalysis – and particularly its Lacanian current – are more wedded to politics than to psychiatry and are thus in a position to serve as 'carriers' of radical political thought into the psychiatric world, and also in a position to make psychiatry's political struggles more salient to the French Left as a whole. Preoccupation with the work of French structuralist psychoanalyst Jacques Lacan is a leitmotiv of post-1968 developments on the French radical Left and in the anti-psychiatric movement. Having Lacan in common has facilitated a certain amount of free circulation of people and ideas between these two worlds.

The 'romantic' wing of the anti-psychiatric movement is particularly interested in the language of the mad, rooted in the world of the asylum, and its concerns fit into a general trend in French radical politics since 1968. The cult of speech which was a part of May (when *la prise de la parole*, 'the taking of speech', was put forth as a privileged form of social action) left a legacy for the Left. Many of the issues which mobilize gauchistes in France since 1968 revolve around groups (prisoners, schizophrenics, children and primitive peoples) which are seen as having special, privileged languages. Indeed, since 1968, the discourse on the politics of madness in contemporary capitalism, the Lacanian discourse on madness as a witness to the 'truth of the subject' (*la vérité du sujet*) and the discourse of French anti-psychiatry have become so interwoven that it is hard to tell where one leaves off and the other begins. This very complex web can be clarified by separating out some of its major themes. Several of them relate to theoretical issues and several to anti-psychiatry as a social movement.

A first theme, one which we have already touched on, centers around Jacques Lacan's impact on anti-psychiatry. Lacan has expressed views which go far towards supporting anti-psychiatric positions, for example, his oft-cited statement in the *Ecrits* that 'Man's being cannot be understood without reference to madness, nor would he be man without carrying madness within as the limit of his freedom'.[3] Psychiatric theory is traditionally based on a 'pejorative' concept of madness in which madness is perceived as a *lack* of rationality, a state of being *less* than what one could be. In Lacan's work, we find the echo and indeed the amplification of all there was in Freud which was most subversive of such traditional psychiatric judgments. The maxim of Lacan's school is a 'return to Freud' which purges normative, psychiatric values out of psychoanalysis. Lacan's return is to psychoanalysis as the science of the unconscious whose goal is the awareness of a level of authenticity (what Lacan calls 'the truth of the subject') which is never confused with an acceptance of social norms.

A second theme, related to the first, deals with how French anti-psychiatry has made contact with political and psychoanalytic currents (among them Lacanian) whose rejection of the intellectual and social *status quo* takes the particular form of demanding a subversive discourse even to state what their positions are. Such people place themselves in a relationship of potential identification with the mad insofar as they claim to have a message which cannot be communicated in ordinary ways. Like the schizophrenic, they have to destroy ordinary language in order to communicate. Some, like Lacan himself, work in a highly controlled intellectual structure and express this identification with the psychotic in a highly theoretical way. Others, more involved in political situations where they are treated as deviant and dangerous, tend to develop a theory of their own situations which liken them to that of the schizophrenic. When groups of people who are not in a classically 'psychiatric' setting begin to identify with the schizophrenic's situation, the social base for an anti-psychiatric movement is being created.

A third theme is the emergence of theories which are inspired by Lacan and which are explicitly anti-psychiatric. Most significant among them is that of schizoanalysis, elaborated in the work of Gilles Deleuze and Félix Guattari, most particularly in their book, *Anti-Oedipus: Capitalism and Schizophrenia*.[4] Deleuze and Guattari, often referred to as the Laing and Cooper of French anti-psychiatry, began their collaboration after the events of May–June 1968. Their concern about the way in which this 'revolution' of speech and desire had played itself out precipitated the inquiry into desire and its role in revolution which turned into *Anti-Oedipus.*

Deleuze and Guattari's study of desire in the social field brings us to a fourth theme, that of the relationship between Marxism and psychoanalysis in France. French anti-psychiatry is both 'psychoanalytic' and deeply embedded in a Marxist tradition of political action on the French Left. The problem of how to reconcile Marxism and psychoanalysis has structured much of twentieth-century social thought. Some 'solutions' to this problem reinterpret psychoanalysis to make it more compatible with Marxism, others reinterpret Marxism for greater compatibility with psychoanalysis. In France there are powerful efforts on both sides with Lacanism moving closer to Marxism and several branches of Marxist thought, some associated with the gauchiste non-Communist Left and some with the French Communist Party moving closer to psychoanalysis. We shall examine both sides of this *rapprochement*, stressing the ways in which it is facilitated by Lacan's very particular brand of psychoanalytic thought.

But the interrelations among French psychoanalysis, psychiatry and radical politics go beyond theory construction to social action. Indeed, part of what makes the French psychoanalytic and anti-psychiatric scenes so special is not only their involvement with each other but their political involvements in a variety of social and institutional settings. Anti-psychiatric and radical psychoanalytic ideas have been picked up by various groups in France, ranging from working-class nurses who are organizing in provincial psychiatric hospitals to Parisian intellectuals who relate to Lacan and his circle in terms of radical chic. In fact, there is both an 'official' anti-psychiatry (that which is written about, that which the intellectuals have picked up) and an 'unofficial', grass roots and anti-psychiatric movement.

Much of the actual activity in anti-psychiatry had its roots during the 1968 events, when many people involved in psychiatry became sensitized to politics at the same time that many people involved with radical politics became sensitized to the political issues below the surface of medical and psychiatric practice. This second group had its desires for political change frustrated during 1968 and turned much of their political energies towards the politics of medicine and psychiatry. They tended to see action on medical and psychiatric issues as important, both for themselves, and as catalysts for what might ultimately be larger political actions. They brought into anti-psychiatric politics the same techniques of organization-building and use of journalism that they had used to build support for other political issues in the pre-May period.

Because of the free circulation of people between the political, psychoanalytic and anti-psychiatric worlds since 1968, many of the quarrels among psychoanalysts (pro- and anti-Lacan) and among political people on the Left (pro- and anti-Communist) have gotten played out in the politics of anti-psychiatry. For example, there are four orthodox 'Freudian' psychoanalytic societies and their positions on psychoanalytic issues tend to have implications for the stands that their members take on political ones. The lines of cleavage on political issues between the analytic societies are not always clear, but a few very marked patterns have emerged in the way in which Lacan's challenge to the notion of 'treatment' and 'cure' tends to work itself out in institutional practice as a challenge to a notion of therapeutic *re-plâtrage*, the masking of social problems as psychiatric ones. Here we shall simply give a flavor of what psychoanalytic politics looks like by indicating how it was played out in the sectors (catchment areas) of the French community mental health movement.

After 1968, when the *sectorisation* program became official national health policy, institutions which would respond to what seemed to be a new level of demand for psychotherapy proliferated in the public sector and became a major source of employment for young analysts. Different centers came under the control of different branches of the psychoanalytic movement. In some of the centers which came under the control of the Lacanian group (that is, whose medical director belonged to the Freudian School) the analysts used the centers as bases from which to challenge their medical and pedagogical ideologies. Indeed, the institutions became places in which Lacan's notions were concretized in an attack on the repressive role of the therapeutic institution on society. Centers that were under more traditional psychoanalytic tutelage, such as those in the 13th *arrondissement*, kept traditional medical orientations. The state health system was divided into psychoanalytic-political units with radically different kinds of functioning. They developed an increasingly charged politics both within the institution and in relationship to the outside (to the social security system, to parent groups and labor unions). Thus, after tracing out some of the major theoretical strands which weave together contemporary French psychoanalysis, anti-psychiatry and the French Left, we shall look at how these theoretical positions have been expressed in anti-psychiatric activity which is often as schismatic as the psychoanalytic and political movements which are its touchstones.

Jacques Lacan and psychoanalysis as subversion

For many French analysts, Jacques Lacan has served as a bridge between political activism and that of a specifically anti-psychiatric variety. Among psychoanalytic theorists Lacan has perhaps gone furthest in his writing to distinguish psychoanalysis from a medical or psychiatric technique centered on a notion of cure or adaptation and to bring it into sharper focus as a process of knowledge-seeking. Lacan has spent his career attacking the American psychoanalytic tradition which he sees as adaptationist and bureaucratized. For Lacan, psychoanalysis is a calling, a process of growth and discovery that has nothing to do with belonging to the bureaucracy of an analytic institute, achieving a certain kind of academic degree or following a series of set rules about how to conduct analytic sessions. Lacan has institutionalized these beliefs in his own psychoanalytic school, the Freudian School of Paris (L'Ecole Freudienne de Paris), where there are not only no requirements for admission (such as an M.D. or a Ph.D.) but there is no set program for becoming an analyst. For Lacan, when it comes to analytic training or when it comes to how to do analysis, the only rule is that there should be no rules.

Many French analysts seem to feel that Lacan and his work are offering them some respite if not relief from the 'American dilemma' of analytic acceptability (what does psychoanalysis become when it is no longer considered marginal or threatening, but rather is considered the 'thing to do') by bringing them back to a vision of what is subversive in the analytic vision. Lacan supports anti-psychiatric perspectives by his criticism of hierarchies and rules that he feels have no place in work of an analytic order. He attacks the idea that one can be true to the Freudian discovery by institutionalizing psychoanalysis in rigid training structures or by following a technique aimed at strengthening the ego. Lacan believes that with its 'routinization', psychoanalysis ceases to be psychoanalysis and there is no coherent ego to be strengthened.

Lacan's contribution to French anti-psychiatric thought comes largely through his radical critique of theories of the ego. In his own work he demonstrates that the ego was formed by a composite of false and distorted introjections so that 'I' and 'Other' are inextricably confused in the language of the self and that any comforting, pleasant sense of the coherence of the self is purely illusory. Lacan's work, unlike some of the writings of R. D. Laing, never becomes an apologia for madness. For Lacan, madness is not the negation of normality with normality defined as bad and madness as privileged or as an 'absolute' good. Madness is quite simply a kind of communication or expressed demand. Because the psychotic has not fully acceded to communication, the Symbolic dimension, the order of language and society, his communications are difficult to decipher.

When we enter the Symbolic dimension, we become subject to its laws of signification, indeed, we become inhabited by them. This is what Lacan means when he says that 'the unconscious is structured like a language', that man is 'decentered'. For Lacan, like Lévi-Strauss, man is the object of a Law which transcends him. Lévi-Strauss'

Indians cannot recognize the rules which govern the marriages between cousins and since Freud wrote *The Interpretation of Dreams* it has been clear that man is inhabited by a Law which he doesn't constitute but which constitutes him. He is inhabited by the Signifier, he didn't create it. Lacan made the decentered subject the focus of his research on the status of human discourse in psychoanalysis and, indeed, on the status of human discourse in general. For Lacan, the resolution of the Oedipal crisis marks the entrance of the subject into the discourse of language and society which he refers to as the Symbolic dimension. We enter the Symbolic dimension by accepting our father's rules and interdictions and, through him, we accept social laws and social language which begin to live within us as presences.

When Lacan speaks of the status of human discourse and speaks of the Symbolic and its law of language and society he calls into question the idea as an entity with autonomy and free will. Lacan believes that this challenge to the Cartesian notion of the subject was one of Freud's central concerns. Lacan's view of the decentered subject opposes that of both the existentialists who focus on the *cogito* and on man's freedom, and that of ego psychologists who tend to speak of the ego as an active, autonomous unity. Lacan's Freudian structuralism undermines the idea of a coherent ego from the time of its foundation in the mirror stage of development.

Since Lacan's notion of the decentered self is so crucial to the appropriation of psychoanalysis into an anti-psychiatric and Marxist discourse it seems appropriate to pause on its origin in the mirror phase. For Lacan, the origins of the self are imaginary, remote from any notions we might have of 'reality'. The baby is fascinated by the human forms around him and identifies with them as he identifies with his own image in the mirror. Thus the person first sees himself in another, mother or mirror, and the primary identification of self is not a recognition, but a misrecognition which constrains all later construction of the self to a state of alienation: the self is always like another. 'The mirror identification situates the existence of the *ego*, before its social determination, in a fictional direction, which will always remain irreducible for the individual alone.'[5]

Since the self is formed from a composite of introjections based on misrecognitions, it can hardly be seen as a 'unified' personality. Thus, even for 'normal' people, the ego is not a coherent unity. According to Lacan we all experience a profoundly 'divided self'. Lacan's ideas about the self seem resonant with those of R. D. Laing but the differences are crucial. For Laing, the newborn needs reassurance and needs to be seen, but it is already an entity and seems to have an essential self. For Lacan, things are altogether different: the baby knows only a subjectibility. During the mirror phase, the child identifies itself as what it sees. Only later will this 'me' be brought gradually, but never completely, into line with the subjective, with the 'I'.

In calling the integrity of the 'I' into question, Lacan challenges assumptions which are solidly built into 'ordinary' thought and 'ordinary' languages. In fact, it is almost impossible to express such a radically 'anti-ego' theory in ordinary language. The language's pronoun structure (I, you, he, she) reflects our culturally embedded notions about our subjectivity. They are Cartesian. From the moment that we begin to write or speak we are trapped in formulations such as 'I want', 'I do', 'I desire'. Lacan's reading of psychoanalysis is subversive in the way it undermines the formulations of the self which are implicit in our language and puts each speaking subject in an intimate relationship with the fragmented self experienced by the schizophrenic. Thus, the notion of the decentered subject is a crucial link between Lacan and the anti-psychiatric movement which refuses a view of madness as something completely alien to 'normals'.

This essay cannot of course be a primer in Lacan's thought, but the intention here is to highlight how his notion of the decentered subject has supported anti-psychiatric perspectives. Maud Mannoni's work represents an anti-psychiatric position inspired by Lacan's work on the decentered subject. Like Lacan, Mannoni abhors any notion of psychoanalysis as emotional reeducation – it is a study of desire and the 'logic of the unconscious'.[6] Although Laing works with the child's role in the mother's fantasy, Mannoni takes this idea further, using Lacan's theories to analyze the child's symptoms in terms of the parent's desires. Laing displaces illness from the patient to the family constellation, but Mannoni goes beyond the patient's intersubjective relations to his language – a framework which the child enters at birth but which is shaped long before his birth.[7] Elements of the parent's linguistic discourse do not allow the child to accede to words of his own. Through the Oedipus complex, with the introduction of the Symbolic dimension, the child can develop a symptom which is the signifier for an unsolved problem of the parents in regard to their own parents.

In Lacan's case, the support for anti-psychiatry comes from the *form* of Lacan's writing as well as from its content. Lacan refuses to write on the 'university' level of discourse that we normally associate with psychoanalytic exposition. His associative, poetic style is intended not simply to shock or to force a closer reading by slowing the reader down, but more importantly, to challenge common-sense notions of the 'self'. This style is shared by mány of his adepts and, indeed, the question of style emerges as an important strategy for anti-psychiatric as well as radical political exposition.

Anti-psychiatry and linguistic subversion

Our everyday language reinforces our 'common-sense' understanding of our experience as subjects. Theories of the mind which want to subvert our usual way of thinking about ourselves must adopt strategies to fight the normalization which language imposes. A first possible strategy is to make mathematical models which in our culture are acceptable ways of 'setting up one's own language'. Any reader who has so much as glanced through the *Ecrits* will surely not need to be reminded that Lacan's work is studded with such 'formalizations'. He uses symbols, signs, charts and diagrams of his own invention to express himself without reference to the symbol system of ordinary language. Indeed, in recent years Lacan has tended to rely ever more heavily on this solution, and in his seminar has emphasized new symbolizations, such as knots and mathematical models of psychoanalytic theory which he refers to as *mathèmes*.

A second strategy is to use ordinary language in a heavily nonconventional way. Lacan relies heavily on punning and word games. He also coins words which have no definitions other than his own and then tends to define them only contextually. Even when Lacan borrows from other disciplines what might superficially seem to be standard technical terms, he uses them in ways where their normal definitions are not applicable.[8] A third strategy involves the invention of a new level of discourse, indeed the attempt to create a new kind of discourse altogether. The idea of using a new kind of discourse to break the reader's usual 'set' is not an uncommon strategy for subversive intellectual movements of the twentieth century. It characterizes the work of Wittgenstein, Joyce, and the surrealists, as well as that of Lacan. In each of these cases, the text is not there simply to transmit content or to convince you of an argument, but *to do something to* the reader. The function of the text is not to replace one form of knowledge by another, but to reject standard notions about the nature of knowing. Wittgenstein takes up this idea in the *Tractatus* where he compares his work to a ladder which is to be discarded after the reader has used it to reach a new level of understanding.[9] Similarly when Lacan gives his seminar in Paris, he claims to be putting himself in the place of the analysand and putting his audience in the role of his analysts. His spoken 'texts' and his written statements are designed to provoke the listener or the reader into a self-analytic experience.

There is a similar 'therapeutic' intent operant in Gilles Deleuze and Félix Guattari's *Anti-Oedipus* which became something of an anti-psychiatric *cause célèbre* in Paris in 1972–3. Guattari is a Marxist activist and a practicing Lacanian psychoanalyst who works at France's best-known 'anti-psychiatric' facility, the Clinique de la Borde at Cour-Cheverny. Deleuze is a philosopher, with a particular interest in meaning and literary production.

Let us look at what confronts the reader when he opens to the first page of *Anti-Oedipus*:

Chapter 1. The Desiring-Machines

It is at work everywhere, functioning smoothly at times, at other times in fits and starts. It breathes, it heats, it eats. It shits and fucks. What a mistake to have ever said *the* id. Everywhere *it* is machines – real ones, not figurative ones: machines driving other machines, machines being driven by other machines, with all the necessary couplings and connections. An organ-machine is plugged into an energy-source-machine: the one produces a flow that the other interrupts. The breast is a machine that produces milk, and the mouth a machine coupled to it. The mouth of the anorexic wavers between several functions: its possessor is uncertain as to whether it is an eating-machine, an anal machine, a talking-machine, or a breathing-machine (asthma attacks). Hence we are all handymen: each with his little machines: for every organ-machine, an energy-machine: all the time, flows and interruptions. Judge Schreber has sunbeams in his ass. *A solar anus*. And rest assured that it works: Judge Schreber feels something, produces something, and is capable of explaining the process theoretically. Something is produced: the effects of a machine, not mere metaphors.[10]

In *Anti-Oedipus* we are presented with an image of a world where complexity and fluidity seem to defy language and its structure. This discourse assaults, the language tries to break language apart, fragment all person-markers and transform the reader's way of thinking about his personhood. Much of the book's power for the reader is due to a level of involvement with its language which has little to do with giving assent to the book's individual propositions.

Lacan believes that the unconscious is structured like a language and that its elements and its relations can be diagrammed, indeed even mathematically expressed. In the form as well as the content of *Anti-Oedipus*, Deleuze and Guattari challenge the notion of one-to-one relationships between determinate objects and, in doing so, frame a challenge to psychoanalysis. The crux of their argument centers around the role of Oedipus complex. Freud's position about the actors involved in Oedipus seems fairly clear: the Oedipal drama which results in the internalization of a parental super-ego is played out in a triangle of child, father and mother. For Lacan, Oedipus is not about a moment in the family drama or about forming a new psychical entity. It is about the child's development of a new capacity for using symbols as signifiers, what Lacan refers to as entering the Symbolic dimension.

According to Lacan, the passage into the Symbolic dimension does involve an interdiction (the father denies the child access to the mother), but the interdiction is not to be understood on a literal level. What is important is that when the child accepts the father's authority and his name, he accepts the Law of signification.[11] We do injustice to Lacan's notion of the 'father' if we think of him in terms of his biological incarnation. His crucial role is played on the level of signification, just as Lacan stresses that the meaning of the Phallus from a psychoanalytic point of view relates to its symbolic role rather than its biological substance. For Lacan, the triangle in Oedipus is to be taken in a very generalized sense; its participants are not people but symbolic functions. What is necessary for passage into the Symbolic dimension are certain structural conditions that are associated with Oedipus and, most importantly, the notion of triangulation.

Deleuze and Guattari relate to Lacan as practically the only psychoanalyst worthy of being disagreed with, but criticize him for remaining with the family metaphor and the notion of one-to-one relationships in the discussion of the unconscious. They mount their attack on the notion of Oedipus.

Psychoanalysis is like the Russian Revolution; we don't know when it started going bad. We have to keep going back further. To the Americans? To the First International? To the secret Committee? To the first ruptures, which signify renunciations by Freud as much as betrayals by those who break with him? To Freud himself, from the moment of the 'discovery' of Oedipus? Oedipus is the idealist turning point.[12]

Their picture of the unconscious will not fit into the Oedipal triangulations whether the elements being triangulated are literal parents or Lacan's more abstract symbolic elements. Lacan criticizes biologism in psychoanalysis, but for Deleuze and Guattari the more fundamental problem is the way in which any notion of Oedipus implies restrictions on a field (the unconscious) where things are infinitely open.

Free association, rather than opening onto polyvocal connections, confines itself to a univocal impasse. All the chains of the unconscious are biunivocalized, linearized, suspended from a despotic signifier. The whole of desiring-*production* is crushed, subjected to the requirements of *representation*, and to the dreary games of what is representative and represented in representation. And there is the essential thing: the reproduction of desire gives way to a simple representation, in the process as well as theory of the cure.[13]

Deleuze and Guattari see man as constituted by desiring-machines: 'The desiring-machines pound away and throb in the depths of the unconscious: Irma's injection, the Wolf Man's tick-tock, Anna's coughing machine, and also all the explanatory apparatuses set into motion by Freud, all those neuro-biological-desiring-machines.'[14] An infinite variety of relationships are possible among the desiring-machines. The model of what happens in relationships is not that one person relates to another whole person, but of interrelations between partial subjects. Each person's machine parts can plug and unplug with the machine parts of another. There is no self, only the cacophony of desiring-machines; fragmentation is universal; it is not the 'burden' of the schizophrenic. But capitalist economic and social arrangements cannot tolerate the varieties of possible relationships and impose constraints on which ones are allowed. Psychoanalysis is trapped in capitalism's notions of the family and sexuality. These notions are constricted and constraining: they twist and distort the production of desire.

Thus, for Deleuze and Guattari the ego is a capitalist construct; capitalist social systems make a self-contained or 'private individual' with a sense of an autonomous *self* just as they make the nuclear, atomized family and private property. In place of psychoanalysis, which they see as the therapeutic modality of capitalism, Deleuze and Guattari substitute schizoanalysis. They feel that schizoanalysis has the potential to release the individual from the constraints of capitalist family structure and from the notions of relations between people being relations of a One to another One. The idea of schizoanalysis, now an important concept in French anti-psychiatric writing, becomes clearer when examined in the context of the more general argument of *Anti-Oedipus*.

Anti-Oedipus as anti-psychiatric theory

Deleuze and Guattari's main thesis is that the focus on the Oedipal triangle of psychoanalysis relates to the social, political and religious forms of domination in modern societies. Their criticism of anti-psychiatric authors such as Laing and Cooper is that they look at the libido within the confines of an intrafamilial communication system instead of realizing that Oedipization is a social-political technique for turning desire back onto the family. In *Anti-Oedipus*, desire takes its place in the ensemble of Marx's forces of production as an element in the social field, not only in the individual psyche. Despotism and Fascism can express desire in the social field – they can also be examined in terms of what Deleuze and Guattari call the individual's 'micropolitics of desire'.

Deleuze and Guattari's thesis is that psychoanalytic theory is complicit with how capitalism has constructed the family because it reduces all production of desires to the level of a relationship between child and parents. Psychoanalysis helps to force our discourse about ourselves into what Deleuze and Guattari refer to as the 'papa-mama matrix' whereas, in fact, the individual's unconscious is not determined by a closed family system, but by an historical-political situation. Whereas psychoanalysts might analyze May–June 1968 in terms of an unresolved Oedipal complex (that is, in relationship to things happening in the family), Deleuze and Guattari would analyze the individual and family in terms of the desires expressed during May.

Deleuze and Guattari develop their analysis of the relationship between the Oedipized family and the needs of capitalist society through an anthropology of entropy, not dissimilar to that suggested by Claude Lévi-Strauss. Desiring machines can be coded and decoded. Coding puts information about the society and its shared social language into place; decoding decreases social information. Decoding represents an increase in entropy (disorder) and it results in society's losing control of the machines' interconnections (their 'flux'). The absolute limit of decoding is schizophrenia. Deleuze and Guattari analyze the history of human society in terms which suggest that as society has moved from a primitive state through barbarian times to the civilized (capitalist) state, the level of code in the desiring machines has dramatically diminished.[15] Society struggles against this progressive loss of shared social meaning, since it would be destroyed by total decoding (schizophrenia). One of its ways of fighting against threatening disorder is to construct the family as an artificially 'reterritorialized' unit in which older forms of social organization (with less disorder) can be replicated. The father, for example, becomes a residual despot, the mother becomes an image for land, earth and country, and the person becomes a 'privatized subject'. This is the subject which psychoanalysis studies within the Oedipal family unit – a construct whose role is to mask disorder.

Thus psychoanalysis, when tied to a notion of Oedipus is not in a position to analyze desire on the level of the desiring-machines in their relation to the social-historical situation. For this, another model is needed. Deleuze and Guattari suggest schizoanalysis (a process of decoding or schizophrenization) whose aim is to analyze how the social field is invested with unconscious desire. Deleuze and Guattari recognize that schizoanalysis resembles curing rituals in primitive societies where diagnosis and treatment involve a political, social and economic analysis of the community and its neighbors and describe such cures as 'schizoanalysis in action'.[16]

Deleuze and Guattari place schizoanalysis at a higher level of theory than psychoanalysis. Psychoanalysis is subsumed by schizoanalysis. In principle, psychoanalysis can unmask contradictions between preconscious and unconscious desires, but this is the point at which psychoanalysis reaches a dead end because it is only able to understand such contradictions in terms of the individual's personal (Oedipal) history. From the point of view of *Anti-Oedipus*, this can only be a contradiction in terms because the Oedipus mythology is designed to hide, not analyze, the contradictions of desire in society. You can't understand something by a process which contributes to its camouflage.

The fact that psychoanalysis is subsumed by schizoanalysis means that schizoanalysis can be used to analyze psychoanalysis itself. Schizoanalysis sees psychoanalysis as caught in a conflict between its preconscious interest to decode and analyze and a contradictory unconscious desire to deny the partial, 'molecular' level of the desiring-machines in favor of a 'molar' level, the level of the organism, in short, the level of 'the person'. Thus, psychoanalysis represses the molecular reality to concentrate on a molar construct, 'the whole person', which is a fiction. By insisting that desire resides in 'the person', psychoanalysis denies the presence and power of desire in the social field, thus reducing much social conflict to the level of individual conflict.

Of course, the essential roots of this misplaced humanism are in the psychoanalytic allegiance to Oedipus. Deleuze and Guattari criticize much of anti-psychiatry for sharing this same allegiance. They attack Gregory Bateson's studies on schizophrenegenesis as 'American familialist' because he claims to have found schizophrenegenic *social* mechanisms at the same time that he claims to have found them within the order of the *family*, 'which both social production and the schizophrenic process escape'.[17] After their attack on Bateson they turn to R. D. Laing:

> This contradiction is perhaps especially perceptible in Laing, because he is the most revolutionary of the anti-psychiatrists. At the very moment he breaks with psychiatric practice, undertakes assigning a veritable social genesis to psychosis, and calls for a continuation of the 'voyage' as a process and for a dissolution of the 'normal ego', he falls back into the worst familialist, personological, and egoic postulates, so that the remedies invoked are no more than a 'sincere corroboration among parents', a 'recognition of the real persons', a discovery of the true ego or self as in Martin Buber. Even more than the hostility of traditional authorities, perhaps this is the source of the actual failure of the anti-psychiatric undertakings, of their co-option for the benefit of adaptational forms of familial psychotherapy and of community psychiatry, and of Laing's own retreat to the Orient.[18]

So even the anti-psychiatrists remain bogged down in a familialism which brings everything, including schizophrenia, back to the Oedipal Holy Family: 'Daddy-Mommy-Me'. Laing may see schizophrenia as rooted in the family, but Deleuze and Guattari prefer to analyze its potential to decode as a process which undoes the family. The schizophrenic exists in an extended network of social forces and his language makes the connections between self and social network more transparent to us. In the schizophrenic discourse we see 'Daddy-Mommy and Me' in relation to race, class, police repression, May 1968, rape, the Vietnamese war. Deleuze and Guattari suggest that through a process of schizophrenization we can begin to see these connections for ourselves as we reject the false coherence of the 'molar' self and experience the self on the level of the desiring-machines. At present, we can either Oedipize and neuroticize or refuse Oedipization and become what psychiatry labels as schizophrenic. Schizophrenization will be a third alternative, distinct from nosological schizophrenia because, far from being out of control, its delirium will be focused on finding the truth of subjectivity and on the personal understanding of the micro-politics of desire.

Deleuze and Guattari describe this process of schizophrenization in ways that recall the language of R. D. Laing. It is a voyage. One sets out to discover the desiring-machines and in doing so, the 'truth of the subject' may emerge. But the resemblance ends with those metaphors.

For R. D. Laing the schizophrenic is on a voyage which is most like a long acid trip. His politics of schizophrenia is a politics of *experience*. For Deleuze and Guattari the schizophrenic's special position has nothing to do with his 'tripping', but is political and structural: he is *'hors du sujet'*, (outside of himself and transparent to himself as subject) and thus is clear to an experience of the desiring-machines of which he is made. As in the work of Laing, he has a higher status than the rest of us, but for Deleuze and Guattari that higher status is political rather than moral or aesthetic. Willingly or not, the schizophrenic has refused the usual manner in which capitalism stamps and controls our psyches.

Thus, *Anti-Oedipus* has several theoretical ambitions. First, to argue that the family recreates defunct political, territorial and social forms in itself in order to mask contradictions in capitalist society. Second, that psychoanalysis, by assuming that all desire is produced in the family, is incapable of analyzing the true nature of desire. It misunderstands individuals and it misunderstands social processes. Third, that if we analyze family myths as a response to social disorder and if we approach the individual as a collection of fragmented, desiring-machine parts, we can move beyond the Oedipal myth which now clouds our self-understanding. This analysis will be a schizoanalysis, 'schizo' because it reveals a truth of fragmentation, the kind of fragmentation that we are used to associating with psychosis. Thus, although schizophrenization is distinct from nosological schizophrenia, the schizophrenic, who has more intimate knowledge of the truth of fragmentation that we shall ultimately discover in each of us, can be our teacher. This teaching is political, not simply spiritual.

Deleuze and Guattari meant their analysis to have contemporary political implications. Authentic political expressions are authentic expressions of desire in the social field. There is no chance that such expressions will come from groups which are constituted by centralized authority structures (such as organized labor). There is greater chance that they will come from groups such as those whose spontaneous fusion precipitated the May–June 1968 events. Deleuze and Guattari call such groups collective expressive agents or subject groups. They come together by fusions of desire and produce and consume their own forms of expression, for example the wall graffiti of May. We can find such groups operating on the large social stage, as did the groupuscules during the May events, or on a smaller social stage, as do groups of patients in a psychiatric hospital. For Deleuze and Guattari, these are the groups to support, these are the groups to watch. Guattari has put it this way:

[They] speak of desire without reducing it to subjective individuation, without framing it in terms of a pre-established subject or in terms of *a priori* meanings ... Analysis becomes political in an immediate sense. 'When saying is doing', the division of labor between the specialists of saying and the specialists of doing is blurred.[19]

The discussion of *Anti-Oedipus* and anti-psychiatry has brought us from issues of form (how style can be subversive) to issues of content which touch on the relationships among anti-psychiatry, psychoanalysis and Marxism. When anti-psychiatric thought attempts to go beyond purely existential categories it must confront its relationship to Marxism. In France this confrontation has been particularly dramatic because the May–June events forced the issue. It was in the aftermath of the May–June 1968 events that a psychoanalytic discourse was appropriated by the political Left and a Marxist discourse was appropriated by the psychiatric-psychoanalytic Left.

'French Freud', Marx and anti-psychiatry

The authors of *Anti-Oedipus* claim that their work closes the old debate on Freud and Marx because it shakes both traditions, demonstrating psychoanalysis' insufficiencies for understanding desire as a social product at the same time as it demonstrates Marxism's insufficiencies for understanding desire in the social field. But far from closing the Freud-Marx question, the publication of *Anti-Oedipus* seemed to recharge it. Interest in the book fed anti-psychiatric involvement with psychoanalysis. Schizoanalysis was read as a political complement to Lacanism. Deleuze and Guattari criticize both Freud and Marx while drawing upon both of them. Unlike psychoanalysts, they refuse to take the 'individual' as a bounded subject for the analytic process but, unlike most Marxists, they analyze society primarily in terms of psychological categories. Their eclectic borrowing from Freud and Marx is not untypical of contemporary French ideological production: French anti-psychiatric theory has gotten closer to both psychoanalysis and Marxism than has its Anglo-Saxon counterpart, a trend which has been facilitated by a *rapprochement* between French Marxists and psychoanalysts themselves.

In the 1950s the French Left, and in particular the French Communist party, strenuously attacked psychoanalysis as an ideology of bourgeois domination. In their own defense, analysts pleaded political 'neutrality', tried to separate their lives as citizens from their analytic work and often denied themselves the political arena altogether. Today, the situation is transformed. Psychoanalysis seems to have something for everyone on the Left. Why the change? It turns out that Lacan's psychoanalytic theory effectively neutralizes some of the complaints that Marxists have traditionally lodged against psychoanalysis. For example, a first Marxist criticism of psychoanalysis was that it 'adapts' people to bourgeois society. This criticism seems to have been disarmed by Lacan's position that only the *perversion* of psychoanalysis thinks in terms of making people 'better'. Marxists face a psychoanalytic movement which claims that, far from reintegrating the casualties of bourgeois society, the analytic process will give access to a consciousness of subjectivity and its limits that can make one a more effective political activist. The belief that there is no apparent contradiction between psychoanalytic and radical political activity is supported by the presence of rather visible groups of radicals who are very vocal about having been analyzed – many of them by Lacan. The circulation of people between psychoanalytic and political circles undermines any notion that depoliticization is an intrinsic property of psychoanalysis.[20]

A second well-known Marxist reproach to psychoanalysis is that it builds up an anthropology in terms of the individual rather than in terms of the political, economic and historical situation. A related point is that in the face of human misery, psychoanalysis treats the individual ego, not the society. This attitude characterized the 'classical' Communist Party position on psychoanalysis which criticized Freud for remaining a prisoner of the dominant bourgeois ideologies of his time. This classical position was best exemplified in the work of Communist Georges Politizer who defended Freud's scientific ambitions while criticizing his lack of interest in history and economics.[21] Following the lead of the Soviet Union, the French Communist Party hardened its position on psychoanalysis during the 1950s, but in the mid-1960s the French Communist interest in Freud was revived by way of the political philosopher Louis Althusser.[22] Althusser, a Party member, put forth the view that the classical Politzerian criticism of psychoanalysis does not apply to Lacan's reading of Freud which focuses on questions of epistemology and the relationship of the unconscious to the structure of language. Althusser and Lacan relate to psychoanalysis as a science and permit Communist intellectuals to look at Freud and Marx, not as social theorists with competing models about how the individual functions in society, but as scientifically homologous thinkers. For Althusser, Lacan's fundamental contribution has been his insistence on the specificity and irreducibility of the unconscious as the constituting object of the science of psychoanalysis, the systematic exploration of the unconscious and of its laws.

With Althusser leading the way, the French Communist Party started to take a more conciliatory attitude towards psychoanalysis, and since 1968 psychoanalysis has been getting a particularly 'good press' in Communist publications, particularly those aimed at the youth movement. Even apart from issues of theory, Lacan's statement in print that the Soviet Union's rejection of psychoanalysis was understandable in terms of how the Americans had distorted it, facilitated a Communist reconciliation with psychoanalysis via Lacan.[23] In any case, by focusing on Lacan, the French Communist Party could emphasize that it was showing its interest in an indigenous psychoanalytic movement, altogether different from that of the Americans. The new Communist interest in psychoanalysis has its own internal politics. The Party is a home both for those who, following Althusser's theoretical perspective, wish to explore the epistemological connections between psychoanalysis and Marxism and for those who feel that on the contrary, in terms of the Party's constituency, it is now most 'strategic' to use a medical model of the psychoanalytic enterprise and to put psychoanalysis to work 'treating' the working class as it has been so long used for 'treating' the bourgeoisie. Given the Lacanian criticism of the American medicalization of psychoanalysis, it is clear that this puts the 'practical' side of the party at odds with the 'theoretical', Althusserian, pro-Lacan group.

Like the Communists, the gauchistes came to their post-1968 interest in psychoanalysis from a position of relative hostility to psychoanalysis as reductionist and as a class phenomenon. What is different is the relationship of their new interest in psychoanalysis to the May–June 1968 events. The Communists disparaged the events and did everything possible to stop them, but for the gauchistes they were a golden moment, and a time during which a direct contact with psychoanalysis was made. During May, the classical gauchiste criticism of psychoanalysis as upper-class luxury paled in comparison with a phenomenal social expression of a desire for contact with psychoanalysts. Wilhelm Reich became something of a *maître de penser*; long nights of political debate were held in a Sorbonne lecture hall rechristened 'L'ampithéâtre Che Guevara-Freud'.

During May–June 1968, psychoanalysts were in demand not just from politicized students in the social sciences and humanities, but from medical students who looked to them for help in creating a new 'human relations' curriculum for French medical schools and from psychiatry students in revolt against their almost exclusively neurological university training. Many psychoanalysts responded to these demands, in particular the Lacanian analysts. The *gauchisme* of Lacan's Freudian School seems related to several factors. There is first the recruitment of Freudian School analysts from Marxist circles around Louis Althusser at the Ecole Normale Supérieure. Lacan held his seminar at the Ecole Normale from 1963 until 1968 when the Dean asked him to leave for political reasons. There is also the fact that Lacan's son-in-law, Jacques Alain Miller, a central figure at the Freudian School, was a Maoist for many years. The gauchiste Left has exempted Lacan from their general criticism of structuralism and seems to identify with his psychoanalytic vision of the decentered subject. In addition to identifying with Lacan's ideas, gauchistes also identify with his behavior in psychoanalytic politics: Lacan attacked the Americans, broke analytic 'rules', challenged hierarchy. For the student movement in the throes of contesting the hierarchy and discipline of the French University system closed unto itself, the Lacanian analysts who had waged these battles within the psychoanalytic world seemed like the officianados of such struggles. In addition, Lacanian analysts had pioneered several experiments in anti-psychiatry (such as that of the Clinique de la Borde at Cour-Cheverny) whose use of 'institutional psychoanalysis' was felt by many to be relevant to the May movement.

Lacan's work has also countered a third Marxist objection to psychoanalysis which criticizes its biological assumptions. Lacan's reading of Freud is militantly anti-biological, shifting all description of sexuality from a biological-anatomical to a symbolic level.[24] This 'return to Freud' returns to the early Freud, most notably the Freud of the *Interpretation of Dreams* whose primary concern is with the unconscious mechanisms of symbol transformation. Lacan insists that Freud never meant to say anything about anatomy and that in those writings where Freud seems to be talking about anatomy he is really talking about how culture imposes meaning on anatomical parts so that they can serve as signifying agents. Thus, when Freud seems to be talking about organs he is really talking about information. For example, in Lacan's models of the Oedipal crisis, fears and desires which others have interpreted as relating directly to real parts of the body (castration anxiety, penis envy) take on a more abstract, linguistic meaning. Lacan's dismissal of the biological Freud makes it possible for French feminists to relate to Freud as a theorist and, indeed, the Marxist branch of the French Women's Liberation Movement is called 'Psychoanalysis and Politics', much to the surprise of most American feminists who are used to portrayals of Freud as one of the great misogynists of all time.[25]

These movements of reconciliation between psychoanalysis and Marxism profoundly influence the French anti-psychiatric movement which is involved with these two currents which have traditionally kept their distance from each other. In fact, the involvement of the anti-psychiatric Left with psychoanalysis is so intense that a movement has started in protest to it. The movement attacks the way in which psychoanalysis is taken as definitionally subversive by the French Left. Its position is well represented by the work of French sociologist Robert Castel. In his book, *Le Psychanalysme*, Castel points out that whereas psychiatry has become the focus of strenuous critical activity by the Left, the Lacanian variety of psychoanalysis is usually deemed untouchable.

Whereas the social role of the psychiatrist is globally challenged, one speaks only of certain psychoanalysts being compromised by power structures which are foreign to psychoanalysis itself; psychiatric theories are completely reduced to functions of control and normalization, but psychoanalysis is simply viewed as having been diverted from what is regarded as its profound vocation; although the purely repressive role of psychiatry is taken as evident, psychoanalysis is simply criticized for having been contaminated by institutions where it has no real role.[26]

Castel argues that when radicals are confronted with evidence that psychoanalysis is complicit in activities which use psychiatric labels to mask fundamental social problems, they tend to deal with this evidence by saying that it illustrates how society 'recuperates' psychoanalysis to use it as an agent of social control. Castel's notion of *le psychanalysme* underscores the ways in which psychoanalysis is not simply 'recuperated' but actively *recuperating*. This position, which finds some support in historian Michel Foucault's work on the history of therapeutic systems, argues that psychoanalysis has inherited the asylum's role of social control.[27] In fact, there is a good argument to be made that psychoanalysis has the ability to take the asylum's policing function and do a better job at it than previous, less subtle techniques.

Psychoanalysis challenges the standard medical division between normal and diseased states and establishes a continuum model for thinking about pathology: we all suffer from the same processes, some of us simply handle them better than others. The continuum model has important social implications because it makes it possible to describe a whole spectrum of behaviors as prepathological, including behaviors which a given society at a given point in time finds bizarre, immoral, or politically inconvenient. Thus, it is not simply a question of psychoanalysis being kidnapped by society to do its dirty work (which is more or less what the idea of recuperation implies). Psychoanalysis carries within itself the germs of its use as an agent of social control. And so, if we look around and find that this is the case, we should not be too surprised. But what is shocking, argues Castel, is that the Left seems too blinded by Lacanian mythologies to take the trouble to look around.

Castel is particularly offended by the fact that the infatuation with psychoanalysis extends to anti-psychiatric circles, whose radical critique of psychiatric oppression is thereby rendered biased and ineffective in fighting real injustices. (Castel makes a special exception of *Anti-Oedipus* which had just been published as his book was going to press.) Castel takes *L'Idiot internationale*, a radical '*anti-psychiatric*' newspaper, as an example of how lack of criticism has been pushed to a ridiculous extreme. He objects that in a 1970 special edition of

L'Idiot internationale entitled 'Against Psychiatry', 'psychiatry is executed without concession, but the references to psychoanalysis are always reverential'.[28] In fact, to add insult to injury, the closing pages of this edition of *L'Idiot internationale* place even the Chinese Cultural Revolution under Freud's patronage: 'This history of man is the history of his repression.'

Castel reserves his most acerbic comments for the way in which efforts in anti-psychiatry which are not framed in 'correct' Lacanian-gauchiste formulas are attacked by the new anti-psychiatric 'in group'. For example, in September 1971, Guy Caro, a PSU militant, was fired from his job as the medical director of the Clinique Burloud in Rennes, a medical and psychological treatment center for students. Caro had attempted to liberalize the center. His experiment was supported by the clinic's patients and staff and even by a popular movement in Rennes. But the Lacanian anti-psychiatric clique objected to Caro because he attempted to do 'institutional psychotherapy' without bringing the relevant theoretical and political concepts to bear. His efforts were denigrated by members of the Lacan- and Guattari-inspired Clinique de la Borde at Cour-Cheverny as a 'patron's pragmatism'.[29] This not untypical judgment from the Lacanian clique provokes Castel's justifiable sarcasm: 'Poor Dr Caro who is only a progressive psychiatrist and a political militant from the provinces and who had frequented neither Lacan's Wednesdays nor Cour-Cheverny weekends: *pragmatisme du patronage.*'[30]

Anti-psychiatry and radical chic

Castel rightly points out that in the Parisian intellectual context, much of anti-psychiatry is really intellectual and social play. The sense of anti-psychiatry as play is reinforced by the romanticism of much of the French anti-psychiatric movement. The group around the Clinique de la Borde at Cour-Cheverny seem to be serious offenders on this score, despite their protests to the contrary. This group includes Félix Guattari, and Lacan-influenced anti(psychiatrists) Jean Oury and Jean Claude Polack. The group at La Borde publishes a magazine, *Cahiers pour la folie*, which specializes in the publication of literature and visual art by mental patients. These creative expressions, while very beautiful, do present an unrealistic view of what life is like in a mental hospital, and indeed of what life is like at the Clinique de la Borde. Mental health workers who work in less chic surroundings were critical of the dishonesty of the *Cahiers*, describing them as 'smug', 'self congratulatory', 'an adventure in surrealism'.[31]

It seems dehumanizing to mental patients to deny the feelings of sadness and despair which they do express by portraying their experience as consistently poetic and by presenting them with glamorized images of themselves in which there can be no self-recognition. Reflecting on the *Cahiers*, one psychiatrist said:

> I know that it passes for humanism, but I find it dehumanizing. I know how psychotics are, I worked, lived among them. They are sad, isolated, resigned, overwhelmed by boredom ... for one Artand, how many patients stay in the hospital for all of their lives and never get up out of a chair? For each Gramsci who writes letters from prison, how many prisoners are completely brutalized, crushed, who think of nothing but the rhythm of the day, the rhythm of meals – because that is what it means to be confined: breakfast is over at ten in the morning and the women stay behind, seated around a table, not talking to each other, waiting for lunch at noon.

It also is dishonest to present a glamorized image of what life is like at an 'anti-psychiatric' hospital such as the Clinique de la Borde. Such presentations are dangerous because they lead to the impression that there are no problems in psychiatry that can't be cured by careful readings and applications of Lacan, Deleuze, Guattari, Polack and Oury. If things are so simple, why should financial and political energies be spent on mental health? In point of fact, the problem of psychosis is far more difficult than that. Although the showpiece of French radical anti-psychiatry in terms of its staff, its ideology, and its spirit and sense of experimentation, the Clinique de la Borde, like other mental hospitals, relies heavily on medication and electroshock treatments in its daily activities. These procedures are not of themselves unjustifiable, but what is dishonest is implying that they do not occur or justifying them in a mixture of Lacanian and anti-Oedipian jargon. It would seem more honest to admit that if we still resort to electroshock in mental hospitals it is because, quite simply, for some people it seems to help, and that, above all else, the tragedy of the psychotic is the tragedy of our impotence and our ignorance of better solutions.

The spirit of play which is endemic in French anti-psychiatric circles seems to have been in some measure picked up from the spirit of the May days which romanticized spontaneity and fantasy. For example, a 1973 meeting at Gourgas was held to facilitate an encounter between political and psychiatric 'militants', but it had less the qualities of a meeting than of an anti-psychiatric 'Woodstock' where the heroes were not rock stars but the stars of the anti-psychiatric establishment: Lacan, Guattari, Oury, Polack, Gentis. Gourgas buzzed with rumors about who might or might not be showing up. In this, the Gourgas experience was not unlike political meetings in Paris whose major appeal is not what might go on but who is there. Even when the favorite celebrities don't show up, at such events they still remain as presences, and the fantasy persists that they will arrive as mystery guests of a sort.

At Gourgas, the festival atmosphere seemed to inhibit rather than facilitate discussion. Participants became bitter when they realized that organizing the sessions meant a lot of work; there seemed to be an implicit contract not to challenge the people who served as the 'mythic' cement for the anti-psychiatric movement: for example, some observers of the Gourgas meeting were offended that the group around the Clinique de la Borde was not criticized for its role in the 'keys' affair of Villejuif Hospital.

In 1973–4, a group of student nurses in Villejuif hospital outside of Paris, one of the most backward mental hospitals in all of Europe, started a newspaper for the hospital's patients and staff. The newspaper carried articles which criticized conditions at the hospital, and it was banned by the hospital's administration. A scandal followed: the Parisian press published a series of exposés on Villejuif. Most notably, a special issue of *Cahiers pour la folie* (dominated by the Clinique de la Borde) and *Recherches* (a journal at that point dominated by Félix Guattari) was devoted to Villejuif. The special issue published the design of the keys to the hospital's infamous 'closed' Henri Colin service. The gesture was dramatic: the hospital authorities had to change all of the locks at Henri Colin. They also fired the group of nurses who had started the newspaper and who were the chief suspects in the 'keys' affair. The symbolic gesture was dramaturgically satisfying, but the nurses were out of a job. Neither the *Cahiers* group at La Borde or the *Recherches* collective around Guattari initiated any support movement for the nurses. These nurses were present at Gourgas, but the whole issue was fastidiously avoided. It is certainly unfair to put the burdens of the whole French anti-psychiatric movement on the group of individuals who work at La Borde, but despite their intentions and their dedication they are a good example of the serious limitations of romanticism.

The events at Gourgas serve to dramatize some of French anti-psychiatry's current problems. Although anti-psychiatry attacks the medical hierarchy, it replaces it with hierarchies based on position and prestige in Lacanian and radical political circles. Although it attacks mythologies of 'normality', it substitutes mythologies of deviancy of the excluded, of revolutionaries, gangsters, and psychotics, all 'outside the law' of capitalist society or 'outside the law' of Lacan's Symbolic dimension. It is undeniable that the anti-psychiatric movement was energized by the events of May–June 1968, but some of May's legacies seem to have been poisoned gifts. Anti-psychiatric 'actions' such as the Gourgas meeting easily slip into 'actings-out' of nostalgia for the May days. Nostalgia and romanticism may be keeping the French anti-psychiatric movement lively, but may also be undercutting its productivity as a meaningful political struggle.

Robert Castel is not alone in his anger at the current state of French anti-psychiatric politics, where serious political issues regarding psychiatric repression have too often become the playthings of an élite which is preoccupied with psychoanalysis, May nostalgia and keeping track of who belongs to an anti-psychiatric 'in group'. In reaction to all of these there is a current of anti-psychiatric organizing which has selfconsciously worked to avoid these preoccupations. It would not be incorrect to refer to it as a French anti-psychiatric 'grass roots'.

'Grass roots' anti-psychiatry

In principle, 'grass roots' anti-psychiatry seems like a redundant phrase. One might assume that a movement which opposes the medical and psychiatric establishment is automatically 'of the people'. In fact, the Paris scene easily supports establishments within its anti-establishment movements. Guattari, Lacan, Oury, Gentis, Polack and Mannoni are a well-published and well-publicized anti-psychiatric élite. Much of grass roots anti-psychiatry is motivated by a feeling that the real political struggle has been abandoned by the anti-psychiatric 'superstars'. The biggest complaint of the grass roots people is that the anti-psychiatric theorists and their showplace institutions romanticize psychosis and show a penchant for prose rather than for the door-to-door organizing that could actually make a difference in the fight against psychiatric repression.

The grass roots efforts center around local organizing and around publications that are less glossy and often more short-lived than those which appear in Lacan's 'Le Champ freudien' series at Seuil or in the

'Textes à l'appui' series at Maspero. For example, the Asylum Information group (Groupe Information Asiles, or G I A), organizes former mental hospital patients into neighborhood groups which are planned so that each group forms a kind of counter-sector. This means that people who were in a public psychiatric hospital together can be in a GIA neighborhood group together when they get out of the hospital. The GIA stresses that when a patient comes out of a psychiatric hospital in France, it is he who is in danger from society, rather than things being the other way around. He has little hope of finding work, the police keep a dossier on him, and if he is ever in the vicinity of any disturbance he has a good chance of being picked up on suspicion. His progress is overseen by his sector's office of social assistance which may inform his employer and landlord about his identity as a former patient. The G I A group is designed to be a support group for the patient and his family and also tries to make communities aware of how the hospital and sector can be socially abusive.

In France, the danger of community mental health programs being used for repressive ends seems real, since plans for the sectors have at various points included such items as evaluating schoolchildren in order to put six-year-olds with 'antisocial' traits into special remedial programs. Combined with the ease with which involuntary commitments can take place in France, the limits on the sector's violation of individual rights seem to proceed from the program's lack of funds, more than from any sense of legal or ethical restraint on the part of the government.

The GIA stresses the fact that when institutional psychiatry invades the school and workplace, it usually leads to encroachments on the civil liberties of poor people: workers and unskilled foreign immigrants. So, for example, projects to administer tranquillizers to hyperactive schoolchildren turn out to be giving most of their drugs to the children of poor people. In short, the victims of institutional psychiatry tend to be ill-equipped to protect themselves. And when these people, often frightened and unsure of their rights, do try to fight back, their efforts are often classified by the medical profession as 'resistance to treatment'. As in the United States, classifying disobedience as a psychiatric problem is one of the most effective ways to neutralize or at least delay a legal or political struggle.

The GIA tries to help 'the psychiatrized' to fight back. GIA programs encourage the psychiatrized to take more responsibility for what is happening to them in their treatment, to refuse to consider it as something which is out of their control. They are taught to 'manage' better their dealings with the psychiatric system by understanding how it works, how diagnoses are made, how involuntary placements in mental institutions happen, how *not* to talk to one's psychiatrist. The GIA teaches patients that maintaining a defensive posture with one's psychiatrists is not a paranoid symptom but good common sense. Psychiatrists rage that this attitude makes treatment impossible, but the GIA responds that if trust is important to treatment, then psychiatrists have to earn it for themselves, like everyone else.

The dominant theme at the GIA is pragmatism. They stress that individual resistance to the psychiatric system is usually punished with the hard-to-fight weapons of institutional psychiatry, but that managing the situation with the support of a group can keep the individual patient out of trouble. Pragmatism also dictates the GIA position on medication. The GIA attacks 'anti-psychiatrists' who take absolute stands against medication: idealizing the 'pure' (i.e. unmedicated) state of madness may make good poetry, but it may be bad for the patient. Since the GIA feels that overmedication is the rule rather than the exception in French psychiatry, patients are encouraged to carefully experiment with modified dosages, but most of the information about drugs that is shared with the patients is designed to inform them about side effects of their medications, since poor patients are rarely told about such things by their physicians and thus become frightened by totally predictable symptoms of nausea and dizziness.

The GIA is focusing its energies on organizing patients because other organizing alternatives, particularly those which organize hospital personnel, tend to leave patients out. If the hospital is approached as one would a factory, nurses and staff are the workers. Using this 'industrial' model puts the patients in the role of the merchandise, the object produced by exploitation, rather than in the role of exploited subjects. It is hard to avoid this industrial analogy for the psychiatric hospital because it corresponds to a certain reality but, unfortunately, this reality is part of the problem rather than the solution. The workers in psychiatric hospitals have low pay and terrible working conditions. When they organize, their immediate interests often do contradict those of the patients. For example, from the point of view of an overworked psychiatric nurse it makes a lot of sense to oppose any liberalization of the hospital because reductions in patient medication and increases in patient privileges usually means more work for the nurse. Thus, it often seems that the only way to change institutional psychiatry is to challenge the entire system or to exploit those few situations where psychiatric workers and patients see themselves as allies and not enemies. This is the strategy behind another attempt at grass roots psychiatric organizing known as Gardes Fous (Guardians of the Mad) which organizes patients and mental hospital workers.

Gardes Fous is also the name of a magazine published by the Solin publishing house. The Solin offices in Paris' Latin Quarter also serve as a bookstore and a meeting place and sponsor for radical health organizations in and out of the Paris area. The locale is a drop-in center for people who want information about such things as where to get sex counseling or a legal abortion, about how to start a small newspaper for mental patients in a provincial hospital, about how to find a therapist whom they can afford.

The project of Gardes Fous is to join together political militants who are interested in the problem of madness with the new group of mental health workers who are starting to see the problems they face in the psychiatric system in terms of a larger political situation. It is particularly interested in fighting against the romanticization of mental illness which it feels has become endemic since around 1968, especially on the non-Communist Left. For Gardes Fous, psychiatry's problems are not on the level of poetry but are about politics.

According to the Gardes Fous analysis, psychiatry uses its cover of medical expertise and 'neutrality' to present itself as offering technical solutions to crises in the capitalist school, family and prison. The army and judicial system use psychiatry to label troublemakers as 'sick' in order to get them out of the way. Psychiatry's value to the ruling class as a subtle, 'scientific' form of social control makes it a good terrain for political organizing.

Gardes Fous is trying to support challenges to establishment psychiatry as they develop in hospital settings. Such challenges have become more frequent since 1968. Psychiatric hospitals have been torn apart by internal battles in which groups of personnel attack the institution. Nurses led the protests at the psychiatric hospitals at Brie, Caen and Villejuif, and teachers, speech therapists and physical therapists have led strikes in psychiatric-pedagogical institutions. Protesting personnel often use what seems to be a psychoanalytic ideology in their struggle against the psychiatric establishment. These protests have been met with the government's traditional weapons: isolation and firing of 'troublemakers', calling police into the institution, and personal harassment. When they are unionized, mental health workers often belong to the Communist union, the C G T. Although the Communist Party intellectuals have latched on to the Lacanian bandwagon, the Party's practical union politics is against movements in psychiatric institutions which shake up the system. So, much of the time, workers are organizing without their traditional union support, and that is where Gardes Fous comes in. The Gardes Fous strategy is to begin organizing on the lower level of salaried personnel in the psychiatric hospital. These workers are *les gardes fous*, the guardians of the mad, whose role in the system is to maintain an order which exploits them as well as their patients.

For a range of radical political groups, psychiatric politics are not isolated from the larger struggles of the workers and peasants who are the *gardes fous*. On the contrary, psychiatric issues are frequently presented as the most appropriate vehicle for organizing them and for mobilizing political energies that were frustrated after 1968. Why? In short, the argument states that in advanced industrial capitalism, the community that was once represented by the state is in dissolution. Citizens are no longer in what used to be the 'normal' relationship with a moral community. Thus, in the eyes of the state, the citizen, *like the madman* and *like the political dissident*, is in a perverse relationship to the normal order. The citizen and the radical have every reason to identify with the psychotic – on a basic level the state relates to them all in the same terms.

Thus, psychiatric issues are in no sense concerns that the citizen and the militant can be interested in but exterior to. The psychotic has gone further than some in his experience of the crisis of the subject, but the psychotic's fragmented experience corresponds to a *'fait de masse'*, a mass phenomenon. The psychotic's symptom is considered as an expression of a socially-shared malaise. By reflecting on the psychotic's situation, the political activist will better understand his own. Thus it is not a question of 'curing' the patient, but of using his situation to shape a societal analysis. The Scription Rouge group, which sees itself as Trotskyist, is typical of groups on the Left which have become involved in anti-psychiatry because it sees Lacan's work as the most appropriate theoretical vehicle for this political reflection.

Lacan never speaks or writes about psychoanalysis in terms of cure. He insults notions of psychoanalysis which see it as a way of 'smoothing over' social contradictions. Lacan defines the subject in terms of its ruptures and crises; for Scription Rouge, his decentered subject is the subject of the capitalist state in crisis.[32] Lacan's anti-therapeutic notion of psychoanalysis is the key to what might otherwise seem inexplicable in the French Left's relationship to psychoanalysis. Because of its impracticality for everyone but the privileged classes, intensive, one-to-one, daily psychoanalysis (what the French refer to as the *cure type*) used to be considered the *most reactionary* of therapeutic interventions. Today, this 'pure psychoanalysis' is regarded as the *most radical* type of intervention. Lacanian 'pure psychoanalysis' is seen as interested in social adaptation. It is seen as facilitating a search for the truth of the subject. It is presumed that this truth will reveal a profound rupture in the state and in the self. Psychoanalysis is thus the highest form of political consciousness-raising and anything else is denigrated as 'psychotherapy' whose goal is to adapt the subject to society. The tables have been turned: classical analysis has become acceptable to anti-psychiatry and the Left.

Many of the connections between Lacan's analysis and Leftist political analysis seem on the level of metaphor. Much of the interest on the Left in Lacan himself seems on the level of the hero-worship of a film star. Although the grass roots movement tries to avoid running an anti-psychiatric movement for the amusement of bourgeois radicals, the 'Lacano-gauchiste' metaphors and the hero-worship reappear in groups which are committed to avoiding them.

Perhaps the greatest threat to the French anti-psychiatric 'grass roots' is that anti-psychiatry is fashionable among bourgeois intellectuals who trivialize it as they support it. People who thought they were participating in an anti-establishment movement gradually find themselves lionized by the Left liberal press, solicited for articles, asked to write books about 'anti-psychiatry from the inside'. After May 1968, student leaders told stories of signing publishing contracts on the barricades. Now it is anti-psychiatry that is news.

The fact that anti-psychiatric issues have been picked up and popularized among the Parisian intelligentsia raises the question of what happens to serious and even potentially subversive ideas when they are integrated into café society. One young psychiatrist who was having trouble in his efforts to get support for the liberalization of a psychiatric service which works with prisoners and delinquents put it this way: 'Refusing to play the game can mean the loss of vital support; playing the game can mean losing contact or real rapport with the people you meant to be helping. They're not following your publicity or going to your cocktail parties. They are too busy suffering. They are in the situation full time, not part time like you.'

The pressure on most people and most groups is to capitalize on publicity and get the support that comes from a sympathetic article in *Le Nouvel Observateur* or from having Jacques Lacan or Michel Foucault say something good about your group to people who matter. Such processes of normalization take place in all societies, but the Parisian concentration of students, intellectuals and ideologists creates a particularly charged hothouse atmosphere where radical thought turns easily into radical chic.

6 Breaking the Circuit of Control

Franco Basaglia*

This chapter describes the events which, starting in 1971, led over a period of seven years to the closure of the Ospedale Psichiatrico in the northern Italian town of Trieste, and to its replacement by a completely new type of mental health service.

This work followed both logically and chronologically on the project which has been described in *L'istituzione negata*,[1] in which a team of workers set out to systematically dismantle the authoritarian structure of a provincial psychiatric hospital in Gorizia, on the border between Italy and Yugoslavia. This hospital was a 500-bed 'total institution' which incorporated all the worst features of the traditional asylum; between 1962 and 1967 the whole apparatus of segregation and repression was taken apart piece by piece – locked doors, staff uniforms, and everything else which maintained the inmate's total dependence on, and submission to, the institution. Many of these changes were parallel to those wrought by the 'therapeutic community' movement in England and elsewhere; but the underlying aim was far more radical. The humanization of asylum life was not seen as an end in itself, but only a first step; the ultimate goal was the abolition of the asylum itself. Thus the project was not seeking simply to make the asylum 'work better', but to lay the groundwork for its total destruction.

The reason why 'perfecting' the asylum was neither desirable nor possible was, as *L'istituzione negata* explains, because its very existence embodied a contradiction – the central contradiction of psychiatry itself, that between *cura* (therapy or treatment) and *custodia* (guardianship or custody). Psychiatry, both as theory and practice, has overtly the medical goal of promoting health, but is compromised by its role in controlling deviance and maintaining public order. In Gori-

*This chapter is based on an address given to the conference on Alternative Psychiatry held in Trieste during 1977. Editing and translation has been undertaken by Maria Grazia Gianichedda, David Ingleby, Pia Bryant and Anna Maria Brandinelli.

zia, over a period of five years, the rules and constraints generated by this latter function were gradually eroded and whittled away to make room for the possibility of a genuine therapy – the recovery of the person, and of the elements of his suffering. In the process, however, the work team ran up against the fact that this contradiction between *cura* and *custodia* was not just a matter of the particular path the profession had taken, but was fundamental to psychiatry as a social institution. It was necessary to look beyond the asylum, at the role psychiatry had in society at large: for psychiatric diagnoses were rooted in the prevailing moral order, which defined normality and abnormality in its own rigid terms; and it was the class system itself which gave rise to the fact that the 'lower orders' made up the bulk of the psychiatrist's cases.

Basic to the psychiatrist's traditional role, and obscured by the aura of scientific objectivity, was the task of isolating and containing social problems and conflicts. This function gave him real social power – the power to single out and classify 'suitable cases for treatment', and to deal with them as he thought fit. Thus, the attack on this system was not just a theoretical critique, but a political intervention – a fact amply brought home by the obstructions and aggravations experienced from the powers that be. At Gorizia, restructuring the asylum and creating a new awareness of the social oppression implicit in 'mental illness' led inevitably to an attack on psychiatry itself, and an attempt to break away from its traditional social function. The project was therefore more akin to the political struggles which broke out in other areas of social life during the 1960s, breaking up established institutions and exposing their shortcomings, than to avant-garde psychiatric experiments like the 'therapeutic community' in England, or 'la psychiatrie institutionelle' in France. And what the Gorizia team eventually came to realize was that as long as their activities were confined within the walls of the asylum, they were at a dead end; it was necessary to go out into the community, since it was there that the contradictions which created mental suffering were located, and there that the drive to exclude and eliminate its victims began. We had to go beyond the world of the mental hospital to confront the madness of 'normal' life: the dichotomies of health/sickness, normality/deviance, man/woman, old/young, which were starting to show their common origin in class divisions and the unequal distribution of power. Health had to be redefined as something other than mere availability for work: and the system which took away from the deviant his basic social attributes – property rights and contractual powers – had to be abolished before he could begin to be 'socialized'. None of this could be done as long as the mental hospital remained the locus of operations.

Hence it came as a logical development in this work when, in 1971, the project of virtually dismantling the city asylum in Trieste, and setting up decentralized community services, was commenced. This drastic restructuring of the psychiatric services was initiated by the local authority in the context of nation-wide demands for institutional reform in every field, and it presented the opportunity of transcending the limitations of the Gorizia project: at last, the abolition of the mental hospital had become a practical possibility. Needless to say, a willingness to experiment on the part of the local authority did not remove the formidable obstacles remaining in the legal and economic systems, and the support for this enterprise from the administration itself was by no means wholehearted.

Moreover, although the team at Trieste was unanimous in its fundamental aim of abolishing the mental hospital, there were divisions here too, both in theory and practice. It must be stressed that this programme was never a matter of simply implementing a plan worked out in advance according to an agreed theory: theory and practice chased each other's tails, and as each new development occurred, the events which had led up to it came to be seen in a different light. Although the fundamental goals were common ones, individual workers had many different ideas about the tactics which should be used to achieve them. And as the identity of the institution was destroyed, so all those inside it – staff and patients – lost their own identities too: all were forced to challenge not only their own practice, but their own understanding of this practice, and the result was a constantly shifting flux in which meaningful patterns could only be discerned long after the event. Moreover, the story of Trieste is really the story of many individual lives, each changing the situation and in turn being changed by it; it would be misleading to describe it simply in terms of changes wrought in an organization.

The common aim in this project, as at Gorizia, was to transcend the medical model and the traditional role of the patient completely, and the abolition of the mental hospital was the nub of this process. 'Mental illness' as we know it was seen not as what the mental hospital cures, but as what it creates: from this source emanate both the categories of disorder and the fundamental meaning of mental illness as something to be segregated and contained. The social fact of *confinement* which the mental hospital enshrines creates a 'germ' or 'infection' which is carried down the line to the private clinic, the therapist's office, and the social worker: as long as the building still exists – even if hardly anyone gets sent there – the mildest form of treatment must conceal the threat of the ultimate sanction – hospitalization. Conversely, to abolish the place is to change the meaning of the psychiatric exercise across the whole spectrum of services, and even in the layman's understanding. Thus the asylum was seen as the lynch-pin of the whole psychiatric system of control, and it had to go.

What about the inmates? In place of their total dependence on the mental hospital, the aim was to re-establish their standing as members of society at large. Patients had to be given back their rights as citizens, both in legal and in economic terms, replacing the relationship of *custodia* by a contractual one. Moreover, this process of laying the unshakeable foundations of his membership of the social body was the first step, not the last, in the rehabilitation of the former inmate. While formerly the institution mediated between the patient and the outside world, the new goal was to establish a direct relationship; to this end, a large part of the team's efforts in the early years of the project went into devising new links between patients and society – job opportunities, accommodation, economic support, and a host of formal and informal arrangements for reintegrating them into the community. As the inmates were discharged, the old system of management which had formerly run their lives for them was replaced by a network of centres in the city.

Let us look briefly at what this far-reaching programme meant in concrete terms. The transformations we are describing did not take place overnight, of course, but over a period of seven years: patients were discharged only gradually, and in the interim drastic changes were made in the way the hospital was run.

The first step was to remove the regimentation and physical coercion to which the 1,100 inmates of the hospital had been subjected. Previously, tight security had been maintained within the hospital, with many doors and windows kept locked; patients moved about the hospital only in supervised groups, to the accompaniment of an elaborate ritual of locking and unlocking doors. They were not trusted with metal knives and forks, but had to use soft plastic eating-implements instead; those who caused trouble could be isolated in cells, or physically strapped down to their beds.

All these constraints were abolished, as well as the administration of ECT and insulin-coma therapy: when restraint was necessary, it always took a personal and not a mechanical form. The staff of the hospital were allowed to develop their own personal style of relating to the patients, with the common aim of establishing a real rapport with them by all possible means, and uncovering the roots of their problems. Drugs were still administered, but solely in order to facilitate the development of relationships and never as a treatment in their own right.

The character of the various activities organized for the patients ('play therapy') was also radically changed. These activities were made voluntary: those which did nothing to fulfil the patient's needs were dropped, and the emphasis was on those which helped the patient to become a social being once more. Important films and plays were put on, which were open to the public and often attracted a large audience from outside the hospital. Theatre groups and painters also contributed to the activities: one project involved building a large blue papier-mâché horse – 'Marco the Horse' – as a kind of mascot, which was then wheeled through the town in procession to the accompaniment of dramatic performances. Holidays were also organized for groups of patients, staying at seaside resorts in regular hotels. Thus, it was not enough simply to remove the *physical* barriers between patients and the outside world: activities had to be devised to break down the *social* barriers which still remained.

'Work therapy', in which a quarter of the patients were participating in 1971, also had to be transformed. Many of these patients provided domestic labour for the hospital, and were paid desultory amounts in cash or in cigarettes: this arrangement was replaced by a cooperative which organized work for both patients and outsiders, on a contractual basis and at decent rates of pay. In this way, the rights and wages given to patients who provided labour were brought into line with those given to other workers.

Of course, the discharged patients could not simply be put out on the street; they still had to be found accommodation and provided for. Some were able to find homes within the community, perhaps with their own families; the provision of welfare payments, given either in regular instalments or in a lump sum, often made this easier. Other ex-patients, for whom this was not a workable solution, stayed together in small groups and rented flats: the idea here was to set up as far as possible a satisfactory community life. In these fifteen 'apartment projects', mental health workers took an active part, but their role was to help the ex-patients regain their autonomy rather than to organize their lives for them. For the majority (80 per cent), however, it was not possible to find accommodation outside the hospital, and to provide for these some of the empty hospital buildings were fitted out as hostels in which ex-patients could eat and sleep as 'guests'. As such, they were not under staff supervision; like the ex-patients who lived outside the hospital, they also received welfare payments, but in their case the amounts were smaller since food and lodging were already provided. Finally, some patients, so old or incapacitated as to require constant assistance, remained in the hospital, and were eventually transferred to the general hospital.

Parallel to the task of dismantling the structure of institutional confinement was the building up of new forms of psychiatric service within the community. From 1972 onwards, the hospital was divided internally into five sections, each corresponding to a sector of the community outside; the total population covered by these 'zones' was around 60,000. The hospital staff were organized into five teams, each responsible for activities within a section of the hospital and its corresponding zone. Increasingly, activities were transferred to 'mental health centres' set up within each zone; some patients were visited by the staff of these centres, but about twice as many attended the centres themselves for help.

The kind of help given by each centre varied, but all were staffed by ex-hospital workers and maintained certain common policies. Firstly, every effort was made to find an alternative to internment as a solution to people's problems: if a patient actively desired to go into hospital, he or she was encouraged to leave as soon as the worst of the crisis was over. Close liaison was maintained meanwhile between staff in the hospital and in the local centre. Secondly, the staff of the centres worked to establish links with other political and social institutions, to spread awareness of mental health problems, and – by organizing talks, films and other activities – to make the centre a meeting-place for the local community.

Thus, although the traditional role of the psychiatric services has been drastically curtailed, in other directions their activities have expanded enormously: although the number of staff employed has remained constant, a large number of volunteers from near and far have contributed to these new activities. A certain amount of what might be called 'psychiatric tourism' has provided some of these volunteers; others have undertaken psychiatric work as an alternative to military service; while many have been psychology students undergoing in-service training. All these outside helpers have been given a good measure of responsibility, and they have made a significant contribution to the whole operation.

As these services expanded and the hospital in-patient population fell, so the need for treatment wards at the hospital declined, until finally only one building was kept open: this unit deals with some admissions, and provides help for the local centres and for the 'first-aid' service described below. (The staff of this unit do not work there exclusively; all have responsibilities elsewhere.) The 'first-aid' team, which was set up in 1977, provides a round-the-clock emergency service: it can be called in, for example, by the staff of the general hospital to deal with situations they cannot handle. The team decides on the spot whether or not to admit the patient; admission is avoided if at all possible, but if it cannot be helped, it is done with a minimum of formalities – relatives and neighbours being contacted in order to investigate the origins of the crisis. The introduction of this service produced a sharp drop in the number of patients admitted to the treatment ward.

The approach that underlies this work is in no way an attempt to evade the central point of illness. In this new context, however, the conflicts which had previously been regarded as internal to the patient, or at least to the asylum, are thrown back on the wider society from whence they came – for the illness is seen essentially as a distorted representation of specific contradictions of the subject in his social relations. For the mental health worker, this means an entirely new role: instead of acting as a go-between in the relationship between patient and hospital, he has to enter into conflicts in the real world – the family, the workplace, or the welfare agencies. These become the new arenas of 'treatment', as the patient's formerly private problems are turned back into public ones. Moreover, mental health workers are no longer impartial: they have to face the inequalities of power which engendered these crises, and put themselves wholeheartedly on the side of the weak. Acting outside the asylum situation, they of course lack any established expertise or authority: thus they have to function without any predetermined responses, on the basis of nothing more nor less than their total commitment to the patient. And while they, in this role, can hardly make a dent in the established power structure whose inequalities are at the root of the conflicts, they gain a heightened awareness of the political nature of people's problems, and of the ultimate link between his work and the wider class struggle.

Once mental health workers have ceased to be an instrument of the ruling class, it is very much an open question what sort of role they can play on the other side, and the team at Trieste has sought to *keep* it open: in particular, it has refused to abandon this mode of functioning for the sake of 'political action' conceived of as something separate and autonomous. Hence the continuous debate among the team – nurses just as much as doctors – over the nature of their work, and the constant quest for new opportunities to extend their role. In many instances, the staff have not waited for programmes to be worked out, but have improvised their own initiatives, dealing with the obstacles in person as they came up. Thus, the process of self-criticism and reappraisal has been never-ending: responses have not been allowed to fossilize, and contradictions have not been suppressed, but on the contrary opened up until they revealed their deepest significance. To do otherwise would simply have been to reproduce the mode of functioning of the mental hospital all over again.

Likewise, even after the demise of the asylum, it has been necessary to ensure that the new decentralized services did not serve the same old function of separating off and exorcizing social problems. To this end – and also to spread the burden left behind by the dismantling of the asylum – the new centres have been set up essentially as meeting-places, where patients and townsfolk could discover their common interests and oppressions. Thus, the services have been set up to minister to the needs of the city as a whole, offering genuine participation and not just paternalistic and coercive 'welfarism'.

Although the cornerstone of the old psychiatric system – hospitalization – has been abolished, the pressure to confine, separate or coerce 'difficult cases' continues to be exerted, and to be resisted by the new services. These demands come from, on the one hand, other branches of the medical or psychiatric services anxious to maintain their own 'efficiency'; and on the other, from individual citizens unable to tolerate forms of suffering which still present themselves as fundamentally alien, and which can only be expressed in the coded form of 'illness'. The aim today is to intercept such problems at an early stage, for example by sending a team into the public dormitory, and by the setting up of the 'first aid' service. Other cases, which under the present laws* would be shunted into the asylum, are simply shunted back by purely administrative procedures. Thus, the channels which traditionally fed the intake to the mental hospital are interrupted at source. The whole tightly knit system is thus broken down, and with the option of confinement removed, the patient's suffering has to be turned from 'illness' into a different form of expression. In place of the old contagion, a new 'germ' is propagated – one for which at present there are no antidotes . . .

It must be emphasized, in case any confusion on this point still remains, that what is proposed here is not mere *tolerance* of mental illness, as the alternative to suppression. When the mentally ill are no longer segregated – conceptually as well as spatially – we are forced to recognize their peculiarities and at the same time to discover our own: for 'normality' can be just as much of a distortion as madness. Only if relationships with the 'sick' person are maintained unbroken can his fellows continue to recognize him as one of them, and to identify their own needs with his.

Although in many ways the project at Trieste might seem to resemble community mental health schemes elsewhere, it is important to distinguish it from psychiatric services which merely reproduce the old contradiction between therapy and the maintenance of public order. Such services are integrated into the existing medical and welfare systems, which are centred on the sanction of *confinement*, and thus they end up by endorsing or themselves employing this sanction. Such services 'work' merely because only the cases they are likely to succeed with get sent to them, and this is only possible as long as the asylum is in the background as a repository for intractable suffering. If we fail to appreciate the widespread ramifications of sanctions against the patient, and fail to take practical action against these sanctions, their continued existence will ensure that suffering continues to be distorted into the stereotypes of 'mental illness'. To leave the asylum behind completely, on the other hand, is not a matter of simply updating the old form of management, or extending it into the community; rather, to take this step is to unmask the system which carefully allocates a measured dose of sanction to each particular case, and to throw into crisis the whole apparatus of social control.

*Since this chapter was written, the laws referred to here have been repealed (see Introduction) [Editor].

7 Report from Norway

Svein Haugsgjerd

In the second half of the 1960s, a discussion took place in the Scandinavian countries concerning the applicability of the model of somatic disease to psychiatric disorders. This discussion was to some extent sparked off by contributions in Anglo-American psychiatry: Thomas Szasz's book *The Myth of Mental Illness*[1], Erving Goffman's sociological accounts, and especially Ronald Laing's powerful synthesis of modern psychoanalytic and family-dynamic views on psychotic states, cast into his own theoretical framework. But the discussion also had its roots in certain components of the Scandinavian psychiatric scene. The psychoanalytic and psychotherapeutic current had gradually grown stronger; combined with the 'therapeutic community' movement and a new interest in family dynamics and family therapy, a broadly *psychological* approach to mental disorders represented, by the mid-1960s, a challenge to the prevailing neo-Kraepelinian academic psychiatry. This criticism of the 'medical model' was also a criticism of authoritarianism and self-importance in the medical profession, and of custodialism and an exclusively drug-oriented approach in the mental institutions.

This discussion occurred in all the Nordic countries, but there are differences in the extent to which the 'psychological' approach succeeded in challenging established academic psychiatry. In Finland, psychoanalytic thinking had considerable influence, while traditional views have kept strong bastions in Denmark and Sweden. Iceland and Norway occupy middle positions in this respect; in what follows, I shall comment only on the Norwegian situation in which I practise.

As a result of this discussion, a change of thinking occurred within the space of a few years – at least among younger members – in the professions connected with mental health work. What was previously assumed to be an assembly of different nosological entities, diseases with as yet unknown aetiology, was now seen as painful psychic states resulting from distressing interactions between people, past or present. The focus of psychiatry was relocated in the interaction processes between the individual and his surroundings – first of all his family, but ultimately his whole social and historical context. Psychogenesis in principle also meant sociogenesis.

This paradigm shift occurred during a period which saw a rapid development of political involvement in the Left among young people. During the early 1970s, public controversy was aroused over certain basic issues arising from the economic policy of Norway's social-democrat government – a policy which aimed at the concentration of capital and resulted in the decline of labour-intensive industries; increasing labour mobility; pre-pensioning of 'marginal groups' of workers; depopulation of many rural districts; urban over-population and anomie, and so on. These issues, heavy with consequences for living conditions and mental health, triggered a strong wave of leftist feelings among mental health workers. This culminated in joint resistance against the inclusion of Norway in the European Common Market, which I shall discuss later. Large groups of mental health professionals participated actively in this resistance, and not only the young ones; in the psychoanalytic and psychotherapeutic tradition a dormant radicalism was temporarily mobilized – a radicalism with roots in the struggle against Fascism and Nazism before and during World War II.

Since 1972, however, the political situation in the mental health field has been characterized by a certain fragmentation, confusion and discord. There are several reasons for this. First of all, the government's policy in our sector has been one of active planning and intervention, aiming at 'modern' institutional reforms along Community Mental Health lines. This new situation, to which we shall return later, has resulted in virtual paralysis in critical discussions of the politics of mental health.

A second reason for the current fragmented situation is the proliferation of a wide variety of professional ideas and ideologies. In the space of a few years, behaviour therapy has become a strong trend within psychology, especially inside university psychology departments. Those involved in family therapy, brief therapy, crisis intervention and so on have largely gone in the direction of 'strategy-oriented' thinking (Haley, Watzlawick and Weakland), which is combined with a polemical attitude against psychotherapy and psychoanalysis. Gestalt therapy has also acquired a following, and an interest in primal therapy and some of the other 'hundred flowers' on the contemporary American scene can be observed.

Certain features of Norwegian left-wing politics also deserve mention here. The largest party on the Left is SV (Socialist Left Party),
ideologically a rather mixed assembly of left Social Democrats and
Marxists of different shades, including pacifist and ecologist sentiments. The smaller but more active Marxist-Leninist party AKP
('Maoists') has dominated among students since 1968, and has also
had some influence in working-class militancy during recent years.
(SV gained almost 12 per cent of the vote in the 1973 elections, and
less than 5 per cent in 1977; the AKP polled 0.6 per cent at both
elections.)

The fact that left-wing politics have almost entirely been connected
with one of these two organizations has had consequences for critical
discussion within psychiatry. In the most urgent political issues –
strikes, for example – the contradiction between labour and capital is
very direct, obvious, and unambiguously articulated. But questions
about the nature of psychic suffering, about how to treat it and eventually remedy it through social and political action, are far more problematic, if we are attempting to relate professional ideas to the basic
contradictions in society.

To make themselves relevant in terms of left-wing politics – and
that also means mobilizing the large groups of leftist mental health
workers in joint action – professional ideas have to legitimate themselves in relation to dialectical materialism and what is currently
understood as Marxist theory of science. Behaviour therapy, located
mainly within the universities, has to some extent succeeded in this,
while psychoanalysis and psychotherapy are generally regarded with
some suspicion in political quarters.

This is a situation which cannot be altered by wishful thinking or
premature ideological efforts. But what I want to do in this paper is
to indicate the direction of my own thoughts, since these are representative of a traditional counter-current in Norwegian psychiatry,
with roots back in the early 1930s when the first Norwegian psychoanalysts were trained in Berlin, partly influenced by Fenichel and
partly by Reich. I want to indicate one direction in which we can move
to make our own professional thinking about mental suffering more
explicit and more comprehensive in its understanding of social and
historical (transgenerational) connections.

As a starting point, I will look more closely at what is implied in
regarding mental disorders as experiential products – as the outcome
of socialization processes in a context characterized by a perpetual

'metabolism of contradictions', and by sequences of transmission of mental pain. In this connection I will make some comments on how knowledge is produced and reproduced in our field. I will then try to show the usefulness of this approach by applying it to the mental health consequences of forced labour-mobility, and to mental hospitals as places of work. Finally, I will outline the argument which underlay mental health workers' resistance to the Common Market, and contrast this movement with the political situation within mental health work today.

Myths about 'the myth of mental illness'

Szasz's title is a phrase that has often been repeated, sometimes with praise and sometimes with disapproval. His basic point, however – that 'mental illness' is a *metaphor* which has gradually slid into a concretism – has often escaped notice in the arguments.

Some protagonists of 'classical' psychiatry saw this phrase as an outright denial of the very existence of incapacitating states of psychic distress. In some parts of the anti-establishment camp, indeed, the critique of the medical model meant dismissal of every kind of thinking in terms of contradictions representing themselves within the psyche. Explanations in terms of intrapsychic conflicts were simply regarded as relics from primeval medical belief; what was wanted were explanations which unveiled social and interpersonal determinants. But however laudable the intentions, a search for sociogenesis without accepting the need for investigating the psychological mediations is bound to end up in a cul-de-sac.

We have all been preoccupied with the immense quantity of psychic suffering in our society. In each single instance, we see how being a human being means right from the start living in conflicts, struggling with anxieties, being at odds with environment and reality. This perpetual succession of contradictions leaves deep traces in us, for each one in a particular way, determining patterns of vulnerability and coping abilities. Eventual mental breakdown in adult life seems to be the outcome of an unhappy matching between the particular strains in the actual life situation and this configuration of traces from the whole process of psychic maturation.

If we are ever to come to grips with the problem of how the sum total and the distribution of mental suffering are determined by the structure of our society, then we will certainly need a theory of the psyche. We need to understand how stressful life events from infancy onwards precipitate 'structures' in our mind – shape, consolidate, or re-shape them. To this end we need conceptual tools, tools fit not only for perceiving, discriminating and organizing, but also for cognitive and emotional elaboration, so that we can become able to tolerate the anxieties evoked by awareness of mental processes.

Psychoanalytic work has brought forward a number of conceptual tools serving these purposes, and will probably continue to do so. To my knowledge, other theories' contributions in this respect are only marginal, even if these theories may be expedients for helping people change.

Professional knowledge as production

In trying to understand more fully what we are talking about when discussing concepts of mental disorders, I will turn to the general question of the formation of theoretical concepts. My position is simply that concepts are tools – in other words, man-made devices for doing some kind of mental work.

As a tool, each concept has its own history. It is invented because it is needed for something: very often it is a modification or improvement of some already existing implement. When a tool is invented, what happens to it depends on whether other people find it useful. Some tools are forgotten, others are copied, imitated or modified. But in contrast to tools for *manual* work, those for mental work cannot be produced by one person and then simply handed over to others; they have to be reproduced in the mind of each new user. For some tools, only a small effort is required for this reproduction, while for others one needs to work tenaciously if the reproduction is to be anything more than sheer forgery.

What I want to put forward, then, is a way of looking upon theories: as sets of man-made tools with traceable histories and specific purposes. This idea is not a new one – it is presented here in embryonic form, and it may be deficient in many respects. The reason why I favour it is that it seems to be helpful in two different problems that have concerned me.

First, it sheds light on many puzzling questions in psychiatry itself: why is it that so many wildly different theories have grown up in this field, going on co-existing without influencing one another and without one winning out over the other? How does it come about that some theories, while explaining so much, are so hard to acquire and reproduce so slowly, while others are learnt quickly, but explain so very little?

Secondly, this perspective on theories seems to be consistent with an historical materialist position in regard to knowledge. By that, I mean a way of looking on knowledge, its acquisition and preservation, in which one is not satisfied with hypothesizing some ultimate categories of thought, defined through some chosen formulations. On the contrary, knowledge about knowledge is really interesting only when one is able to show, concretely and in detail, how some circumscribed conceptual tools have been brought forward as answers to specific questions, at some particular moment in the history of mankind. What kind of need is this or that theory intended to satisfy, and how is this need and this answer determined by the characteristics of the social formation at the time?

Psychiatric concepts as tools

What is striking about psychiatry is the vast number of different sets of concepts, quite unrelated to each other, that have been invented. The explanation of this can be sought through considering the different mental tasks every particular conceptual invention is to accomplish.

To illustrate this, let us go back to Emil Kraepelin, the main representative of academic psychiatry around 1900 and one of the founding fathers of nosological classification. One reason why his work represented a step forward was his insistence on the principle that any sound classification must be based, not on the appearance of the disorder at any arbitrary point in time, but on observation of its long-term development.

Kraepelin's most famous invention was the set of concepts of 'dementia praecox' – actually an improvement of tools from Morel, Hecker, Kahlbaum and others. What is this set of concepts supposed to do? First, it is a device for screening a population of insane people, to single out those whose recovery is improbable. In Kraepelin's own view, this was an unalterable fact of natural history, while we would look upon it as facts of social history – individual fates shaped by a multiplicity of unfavourable psychological circumstances, among which hospitalization was a crucial one.

Be that as it may, why is such prognostic prediction important? I will put it this way: when doctor and staff scrutinize the inhabitants of the hospital ward by means of the conceptual device 'schizophrenia', this serves an important protective purpose. For every patient apparently fitting into this category, a mental reservation occurs, going something like this: 'When making this troubled person a part – however small – of my inner world, I must refrain from every hope that he or she will recover, because such a vain hope, however secretly entertained, will certainly cause me hurt.' Nobody who works in a mental hospital can avoid introjecting the persons who live in it, and the emotions that ensue can be very strong. This is evident, for instance, in those cases where an unexpected improvement in a patient stirs up ambivalent sentiments in the doctors and staff.

Diagnosing also gives other gains. It may furnish feelings of mastery and professional adequacy, thereby preventing discomfort in the company of patients' relatives, colleagues and fellow citizens. It may give inner tranquillity through establishing lines of demarcation between the grossly insane and the not so insane, thereby disposing of worries about one's own madness and perversions. This kind of protective exclusion and projection, very well described by Foucault[2] and Szasz,[3] is of course a very important factor determining the counter-irrationality in procedures for handling the mentally disturbed. But it is only one side of the coin, the other being the restrictions imposed upon one's own incessant activity of introjecting the environment.

Quite a different kind of knowledge is produced within the activities of psychotherapy and psychoanalysis. These concepts are invented for other purposes – they are answers to other kinds of questions.

Freud witnessed the changes happening to the troubled persons who entered upon the journey of the 'talking cure', lying down on the couch and in his presence trying to put into words whatever came to their mind. This setting, called psychoanalytic, presented the therapist with severe challenges: not only of trying to understand the psychic reality of the other person, but also the problem of how to think about the thoughts occurring in the analyst's mind during the session. Thus, the conceptual tools of psychoanalysis serve two purposes: to apprehend the other person's psychic reality, and to think about the thoughts arising in one's own mind.

Knowledge of the psyche is obtained in quite a different way from knowledge in other areas, because the 'optics' for observing psychic events cannot simply be handed over from artisan to apprentice, but have to be developed anew by every analyst-to-be through a painful process of many years' duration. Inevitably there will be discrepancies in perception between those who have gone through this process and the non-analytic spectator. This alone is sufficient reason why psychoanalysis will always be contradicted, accused of epistemological totalitarianism and unscientific circularity of argument, and so on. Psychoanalysis therefore will probably never cease to be a *movement*.

Some readers may ask: what is the point of this preoccupation with the how and whence of psychoanalytic knowledge? I see the future of psychiatry, if it is to be more than just social cosmetics, as very much linked to the future of psychoanalysis. As a worker in a mental hospital, much concerned with psychotic states, their transmission from one generation to another and their relation to the environment, I have been helped a lot by the concepts of Winnicott,[4] Bion[5] and Meltzer.[6] It is my belief that this thinking in terms of psychic objects, space and dimensionalities can prove to be a very good starting-point for new investigations in the transgenerational production and reproduction of mental disorders. In the tradition of family dynamics, the most helpful approach in my experience has been that of Helm Stierlin,[7] with his concepts of binding, delegating and expelling relationships. Eventually, of course, we must understand these processes in relation to the laws of the social formation – laws of exchange, commodity production, valorization of capital and relations between classes; a substantial contribution to this problem has been made, as far as I know, only by Alfred Lorenzer,[8] the leading Marxist psychoanalyst in Germany.

Psychiatry and social history: the case of forced labour-mobility

Ever since Ødegard's pioneering pre-war investigations of psychiatric morbidity in U.S. emigrants compared with non-emigrants and U.S. residents, there has been a strong tradition in Norwegian academic psychiatry concerned with the relation between social conditions and mental disorders. (This fits in with a strong tradition of social history in Norway, largely concerned with the working-class population and written by historians of Marxist orientation.) Apart from Ødegard, many subsequent researchers have made contributions to problems concerning the influence of social and economic factors and stressful life events on overall psychiatric morbidity.

Without going into the issues of these various epidemiological studies, I will simply point out their general compatibility with the conviction growing from psychotherapeutic work: that living conditions really matter – shaping early experiences, determining the amount and kind of life stress and ultimately also the resources with which to counter an eventual breakdown in mental functioning.

As an illustration of how living conditions and social change can be expected to influence the environment relevant for psychic maturation, I will turn to a problem that prompted me to start thinking along these lines.

In 1969, I became occupied with the mental health implications of labour migration, and especially the weekly oscillation between home and work which is common, e.g. in the construction industry. Throughout the 1960s an accelerated centralization of capital and work took place in Norway. There was an increasing flux from the primary sectors of agriculture, forestry and fishing to the industrial sectors, a decline in small-scale production and production based on low-level technology, and a corresponding growth of the monopoly part of capital. Demographically, this meant migration from countryside to urban centres, resulting in the accumulation of social problems in many depopulated rural areas as well as in urban ones. Because of the lack of jobs in the local communities and lack of housing and rapidly increasing costs of living in the cities, a third alternative between migration and staying behind forced itself upon an increasing number of families: the husband working in the city, living in hostels or lodgings during the week and returning to the family at the weekend. When communication facilities permitted, some of these oscillating workers preferred to travel even for five or six hours a day to be able to live at home.

As a physician in a local community where a very large proportion of families lived in this semi-split way, I was struck by the psychological hardiness of many of these people – their bravery and their ability to cope with this extraordinarily stressful family situation. But I also could not escape noticing some of the psychological misery created under these conditions, and pondering upon the possible long-term, hidden costs in terms of all kinds of inhibition of maturation. Of course, living like this has very different implications for different families, depending on a lot of other psychological, social and economic conditions. Nevertheless, some dimensions of family life will be affected, to a greater or lesser extent, in most cases.

For my purpose, it is natural to focus on the parental functions, that is the possibilities for the parents to be 'good enough' as the facilitating environment for the children's psychic maturation. I will borrow terms from the Norwegian psychologist Anne Marit Duve, whose book[9] on the first year of life created strong controversy in the women's liberation movement. Describing the first year of postnatal life as the period of psychological gestation, she refers to the mothering function as the act of gestating the infant through its period of mental immaturity, while the fathering function is described as the deliverance or releasement of the mothering function in the mother.

Leaving aside the controversial issue of the specificity or nonspecificity of the roles of mother and father, I will emphasize her conception of the 'fathering function' as a useful starting-point for a consideration of the qualities of the actual relationship between the spouses that is necessary for each of them to be able to be 'good enough' containers for the infant's anxieties.[10] In the families mentioned above, the husband being away except for the weekends, it seemed that hidden feelings of being deserted by the other, or oneself having deserted the relationship, were frequently present. For husband and wife to start growing to know each other and to modify their original perception of the other, based on projective identification, certain conditions are required which simply were not possible for these families – such as some degree of shared external reality, some amount of time spent awake together as a twosome, some continuity in being together to take the risk of exposing conflicts. The deficiency in marital relationship will, in a large number of cases, result in an inadequate 'fathering function' in either or both spouses, i.e. a relative lack of releasement of the partner's containing function. The consequence, when not counteracted by other propitious psychological influences, may easily be insufficient psychic gestation periods for the children, manifest later in a variety of states of immaturity.

What goes on in the mental hospital?

It is a generalization – but not an unwarranted one – to state that the gross and lasting kinds of psychic suffering, the impairing sequelae of psychotic eruptions or their hidden equivalents, are a plague more likely to fall upon the deprived and powerless: the unemployed, marginal segments of the proletariat and countryside semi-proletariat, people in declining areas of the economy and people whose social origin and education give them few reasons to expect much from the future.

The mental hospitals have been – and still are – the residence of a considerable proportion of our population, for some a temporary, for others a permanent one. Life in these institutions comprises an important but neglected part of our country's social history. Inside this segregated domain of public life, the class nature of society discloses itself in a multitude of ways: in recruitment, especially to the group of permanent residents, in the relations between residents and the public life outside, and so on.

An even more neglected area, however, is the situation of the asylums' attendants. During the last part of the 1960s, in the heyday of anti-psychiatric sentiments among the students of the mental health professions, the custodial mental hospital and its staff were considered almost as a symbol of suppression and authoritarianism. Even today, the contradictions between old-timers and newcomers in the wards are formidable obstacles both to development in nursing and to political work. During a symposium on pre-war working conditions in Gaustad Hospital, the Old Guard presented many vivid descriptions illuminating both the past and present situations. The prevailing unemployment in the 1920s and 1930s was an important factor influencing choice of job. The typical mental institution worker was a person coming from a rural community where opportunities for education and work were absent, and where other people, relatives or acquaintances, had already taken jobs in the same institution. The job was poorly paid, and submission to rigorous and quasi-feudal regulations concerning discipline, housing, leisure time and so on was demanded. Because of the public image of the madhouse, you did not inform other people that you worked there, unless you had to. On the other hand, it did mean employment, after all, and if you behaved well, the job was a safe one. Many learnt, however, to like their work – utilizing their capacity for empathy, getting emotional nourishment from keeping company with the patients, developing self-respect and professional pride.

If we are to approach the mental institution in its full social and political context, we cannot avoid contemplating the particular nature of the work done there. What is a mental hospital?

If we start from our best intentions, we could perhaps say, as some colleagues have done, that the mental hospital should be some kind of a university, where people who have to, can learn something that cannot be learnt otherwise: about regressions, about anxieties, about how to restitute a world to live in after you have experienced a catastrophic collapse in your psyche. The realities, however, are almost always a far cry from these intentions. To be able to extract the ore of know-

ledge – knowledge of what it is to be human – from the rocks of suffering, you need help from somebody who knows something about
this kind of mining. And for most mental patients, such a person
simply was not there.

The mental hospital is therefore more properly described as a site
where immense deposits of mental pain can be found. I choose this
geological metaphor because it conveys so much of my own experience there. When you dig, that is, when you take the time really to
talk to people, everywhere you will find that beneath the surface, distinct strata, sediments of life history and psychic events remain, unaffected by the course of time. These thousands of individual life
histories are not only to be detected in their intra-psychic transformations, however – like reminiscences, reveries, gestures and habits – but
also through what they crystallize in the whole social system of the
asylum: regulations, fixed notions about the management and care of
the mentally ill, attitudes towards expressions of pain, their utter
despair, all are inevitably transmitted to attendants, nurses, doctors
alike. Despite the protective shield of professional roles, our own
psychic state cannot remain unaffected in this kind of work. What
happens is that a large proportion of the pain projected is reflected, as
from a plane metallic surface – hence the harshness of customs and
everyday routines in the wards. This freewheeling of unmodified projective identification can even create effects which may aptly be termed
'counter-persecutory' on the institution's part.

Mental health and anti-imperialism: the struggle against the European Common Market

The most important recent political event in the mental health field in
Norway was the struggle against the Common Market which culminated in the victory in the 1972 referendum. The anti-Market
struggle had been an important issue for the Left since the question
was raised in 1961, but not until 1969 did the anti-Market forces really
grow into prominence. The Left was joined by the agrarian sector of
the economy: farming and fishing regions. The historically important
cultural contradiction between city and countryside, between centrum
and periphery, between urban 'cosmopolitanism' and rural 'national-
ism', was set in motion, doubling, as it were, the impact of the contradiction capital/labour.

The formation of the EEC was perceived as a natural expression of the inherent strivings for maximal capital valorization among the leading strata of the West European bourgeoisie (i.e. the monopoly capitalists of the transnational corporations), an aim to be realized through removing barriers of capital and labour movements. It would also mean a long-term elimination of labour movement resistance to capital's own kind of rationality, since a Brussels-located Common Labour Movement Secretariat could hardly be anything else than a 100 per cent integrated protagonist part of the super-State machinery.

Since the government and Social Democrat Party officials, most newspapers and the key commentators in mass media all belonged to the pro-EEC bloc, together with the Conservative Party and the big bourgeoisie, the resistance gained more and more of the character of a Popular Anti-Imperialist Front, and the emotional climate grew much hotter than it ever has been in post-war Norway. One indication is the mushrooming of appeal campaigns in all branches of public life. One of these was the Anti-Market Committee for professionals in Mental Health and Social Medicine. Its platform went like this:

Until now economy and business have dominated the EEC discussion. People and their living conditions are often forgotten.

In recent years we have learnt that external nature is vulnerable. Protection of the environment is generally agreed upon.

But human nature is vulnerable too. We cannot cope with unlimited amounts of strain. We need a good enough environment to maintain health and continue growing as human beings.

The EEC question is a question of environment. It is important for our mental and social health. Will our basic needs be better met if we join the EEC?

Equally distributed prosperity and economic security are important aims. Opinions differ as to what will bring the highest economic growth – membership in EEC or another alternative. In any event, the difference will probably not be a large one. More important is the question: in what way will this economic growth come about, and how will it be distributed? Joining the EEC will mean becoming part of a larger economic and social system. Basic in this system are 'free movement of capital', 'equal right for establishing enterprises' and 'mobility of labour'. These phrases may sound nice, pretending to equate efficiency, profitability, freedom and equality. But they mean a social reality far from benevolent.

We who work in the health services know that people cannot just be made migrants as 'mobile labour' without causing serious problems.

'Mobility of labour' means families on the move – people whose connections to their environment are ruptured. People will be subject to heavier strain. The 'freedom' will benefit the few, the insecurity will befall the many.

Membership in EEC will imply that economic and technological forces can operate without restrictions across national borders. This means we will have to adapt to the level of economic competition in the larger market. From a narrow economic point of view it may seem profitable to concentrate capital and pursue a rough rationalization in the different branches. But for the individual and his family this often means intolerable stress. More people are forced to move to overpopulated urban centra. Many rural communities will face depopulation, and the local community's social life is eroded. Many are forced to travel too long distances for work, or have to move away from their families. Severe strains or involuntary separations are imposed upon many families. Social and mental health problems will increase.

We know that most people do not wish to be retrained for other kinds of work than their original profession, and even less to be pensioned off before they reach pensionable age. We neither wish nor are willing to adjust to any life situation imposed upon us by a forced effectivization in the economic sphere. For the EEC's one-sided emphasis on economic goals, we will have to pay with increased stress, more mental suffering, more people experiencing themselves as social failures. Those who will suffer most from this are the groups that are already liable to these problems: the aged, the disabled, women, children, people living in rural areas far from the centres, people employed in branches of low profitability, people with little education.

This manifesto – of which the first half is rendered here – gathered 900 professionals from the mental and social health services: doctors, nurses, psychologists, social workers, and so on. It is interesting to note that about half of the psychoanalysts supported the manifesto, even if the reasons for a psychoanalyst not to expose his political opinions in public are strong and well-founded. That so many chose in this situation to depart from this rule is an indication that the issue was perceived as one of immense importance.

The two-year-long struggle in all public arenas had one important implication which can only be seen to a certain degree from the carefully worded manifesto: the relevance of considering social change as determined by the laws of political economy was demonstrated beyond doubt. For all who joined the resistance movement, regardless of the political opinion they favoured originally, they learnt many a lesson on what imperialism is about.

The political unity built among mental health workers during

1970–72 is unlikely to prove long-lasting, however. The new problems facing us today are different, divergences in professional ideology have reappeared as divisive factors.

Mental health, capitalism and social democracy: the situation in the mid-1970s

One characteristic feature in the mental health scene in our country in the mid-1970s is the active, interventionist policy of the State authorities. They show a strong interest in mental health planning and restructuring along community mental health lines. This implies formation of governing agencies on all levels, which means an integration of professional and political leadership. The options of the health authorities, however, are fixed by narrow constraints determined by the Department of Finance and its large machinery of economic planning technology. In this way the professionals are gradually pushed into the role of executives of a policy constrained by cost-benefit calculations. A contradiction between considerations of efficient administration and development of the professional quality of the services offered becomes more and more apparent. The objectives of health authorities are to get the largest 'quantity' of services for the smallest expenses possible. What is needed for an institution or a community mental health centre to develop any 'services' really worth the name, is a problem which is very vaguely understood by planners and administrators. The result of this is a zeal where administrative 'modernizations' and increase in patient turnover is concerned, but a negative attitude towards all questions concerning professional quality. Psychotherapy and psychoanalysis are in some of these quarters considered 'a luxury', outdated if not outright immoral. Helping psychiatric patients should be done through a few techniques quickly picked up by going through some curriculum, techniques whose efficiency should easily be proved through built-in evaluation procedures.

The prevailing climate is a very unfavourable one for joint political struggle in our field. Very easily, people are divided along lines of different professions, different kinds of experiences and different work settings.

A Marxist position goes along the following lines, very roughly sketched: Our country is one where capitalist relations pervade all regions of society. In other words, the bourgeoisie is the ruling class –

the economic and political sphere is functioning according to premises which are the manifestations of the endeavours of the bourgeoisie to maximize the valorization of capital.

The apparatuses of State are vehicles with which the ruling class implements its political hegemony; this also goes by necessity for that part of State machinery that concerns health policy. The class origin of the present mental health policy can be detected when we take a close look at it: it carries a stamp of Taylorism, rationalization and (supposedly) effectivization, disguised by a decorum of anti-custodialism and streamlined modernization. To show this in detail in every case, however, is a cumbersome task. And even more important: psychologically speaking, it is a great leap from joining the anti-imperialist movement of 1970–72 to adopting a Marxist analysis of the State, which involves questions of political identity in quite another way.

The reason why I consider the future relationship between Marxism and psychoanalysis so important is that I think the Marxist conception of social and historical facts is basically true. And it is not only true, but also highly relevant as a guideline for action, because oppression and injustice are predominant in most parts of the world, and for a large part of this oppression, its links to the rule of capital can be demonstrated beyond any doubt.

As for psychoanalysis, I see it as a question of wanting to know what really is in our mind, and accepting that knowledge. A future psychiatry where there is no room for psychoanalysis will mean by and large a capitulation in the face of the real problems of human existence, covered up by pharmacological and game-learning cosmetics.

Notes

Introduction

1. Kiev, A., *Transcultural Psychiatry*, Penguin, 1972.
2. Clare, A., *Psychiatry in Dissent*, Tavistock, 1976.
3. Jacoby, R., *Social Amnesia*, Beacon, 1975.
4. Sedgwick, P., 'Mental illness *is* illness', *Salmagundi 20*, 1973, pp. 196–224. See also 'R. D. Laing: Self, symptom and society', in Boyars, R., and Orrill, R., (eds.), *Laing and Anti-Psychiatry*, Penguin, 1974.
5. Mitchell, J., *Psychoanalysis and Feminism*, Penguin, 1975.
6. Radical Therapist Collective, *The Radical Therapist*, Penguin, 1974.
7. Jones, Maxwell, *Social Psychiatry in Practice*, Penguin, 1968.
8. For example: Berke, J., *Butterfly Man*, Penguin, 1979; Barnes, M., and Berke, J., *Mary Barnes*, Penguin, 1973.
9. Cooper, D., *The Language of Madness*, Allen Lane, 1978.
10. Basaglia, F., (ed.), *L'istituzione negata*, Einaudi, 1968.
11. Habermas, J., *Knowledge and Human Interests*, Heinemann, 1972.

1. Understanding 'Mental Illness'

I. The critique of positivist psychiatry

1. Coulter, J., *Approaches to Insanity*, Martin Robertson, 1973, p. ix.
2. in Stoffels, H., 'The problem of objectivity in medicine', *The Human Context 7*, 1975, pp. 517–29.
3. Kuhn, T. S., *The Structure of Scientific Revolutions*, University of Chicago Press, 1962.
4. Evans-Pritchard, E. E., *Witchcraft, Oracles and Magic among the Azande*, Oxford University Press, 1937.
5. Roth, M., 'Psychiatry and its Critics', *British Journal of Psychiatry 122*, 1973, pp. 373–8.
6. Habermas, J., *Erkenntnis und Interesse*, Suhrkamp, 1968; English trans., *Knowledge and Human Interests*, Heinemann, 1972.
7. Bernstein, R. J., *The Reconstruction of Social and Political Theory*, Blackwell, 1976.
8. Mayer-Gross, W., Slater, E., and Roth, M., *Clinical Psychiatry*, Cassell, 1960.
9. in Giddens, A., (ed.), *Positivism and Sociology*, Heinemann, 1974.

10. Harré, R., and Secord, P. F., *The Explanation of Social Behaviour*, Blackwell, 1972.

11. Gauld, A., and Shotter, J., *Human Action and its Psychological Investigation*, Routledge, 1977.

12. Laing, R. D., 'A critique of the so-called "genetic theory of schizophrenia" in the work of Kallmann and Slater', unpublished MS., 1962. Reprinted in Evans, R. I., *R. D. Laing: The Man and his Ideas*, Dutton, 1976.

13. Robertson, A., 'Sociology and the study of psychiatric disorder', *The Sociological Review 17*, 1969, p. 382.

14. op. cit., Note 1.

15. Heritage, J., 'Assessing people', in Armistead, N., (ed.), *Reconstructing Social Psychology*, Penguin, 1974.

16. Garfinkel, H., *Studies in Ethnomethodology*, Prentice-Hall, 1967.

17. Clare, A., *Psychiatry in Dissent: Controversial Issues in Thought and Practice*, Tavistock, 1976.

18. Torgerson, W., *Theory and Method of Scaling*, Wiley, 1958.

19. Cicourel, A. V., *Method and Measurement in Sociology*, Free Press of Glencoe, 1964.

20. Heritage, op. cit., Note 15.

21. op. cit., Note 1.

22. Heather, N., *Radical Perspectives in Psychology*, Methuen, 1976.

23. op. cit., Note 17.

24. Rosenhahn, D. L., 'On being sane in insane places', *Science 179*, 1973, pp. 250–58.

25. Durkheim, E., *Le Suicide*, Felix Alan, 1897; English trans., Free Press, 1951.

26. Wing, J., *Reasoning about Madness*, Blackwell, 1978.

27. Laing, R. D., *The Divided Self*, Tavistock, 1960, p. 29; Penguin, 1965.

28. op. cit., Note 17, p. 82.

29. Lindsay, G., and Aronson, E., (eds.), *Handbook of Social Psychology 2*, Addison-Wesley, 1968, pp. 61–70.

30. Eysenck, H. J., *Uses and Abuses of Psychology*, Penguin, 1953.

31. Rosenthal, R., *Experimenter Effects in Behavioural Research*, Appleton-Century-Crofts, 1966.

32. op. cit., Note 17.

33. Kamin, L. J., *The Science and Politics of I.Q.*, Wiley, 1974; Penguin, 1977.

34. op. cit., Note 12.

35. Jackson, D. D., *The Aetiology of Schizophrenia*, Basic Books, 1960.

36. op. cit., Note 17, p. 173.

37. See Laing, op. cit., Note 12.

38. cf. Sieger, M., Osmond, H., and Mann, H., 'Laing's models of madness', *British Journal of Psychiatry 115*, No. 525, 1969. Reprinted in

Boyers, R., and Orrill, R., (eds.), *Laing and Anti-Psychiatry*, Penguin, 1972.

39. See Richards, M. P. M., 'Interaction and the concept of development: the biological and the social revisited', in Lewis, M., and Rosenblum, L. A., (eds.), *Interaction, Conversation and the Development of Language*, Wiley, 1977.

40. Heston, L. L., 'Psychiatric disorders in foster home reared children of schizophrenic mothers', *British Journal of Psychiatry 112*, 1966, pp. 819–25. Reprinted in Maher, B., (ed.), *Contemporary Abnormal Psychology*, Penguin, 1973.

41. Siirala, M., *Medicine in Metamorphosis*, Tavistock, 1969.

42. Brown, G. W., and Harris, T., *Social Origins of Depression*, Tavistock, 1978.

43. op. cit., Note 1, p. 40.

44. Foucault, M., *Histoire de la Folie*, Libraire Plon, 1961; English trans., *Madness and Civilisation*, Tavistock, 1967.

45. Baruch, G., and Treacher, A., *Psychiatry Observed*, Routledge & Kegan Paul, 1978.

46. Szasz, T., *The Myth of Mental Illness*, Harper and Row, 1961; Paladin, 1972; *Ideology and Insanity*, Doubleday, 1970; Penguin, 1974.

47. Lemert, E. M., *Social Pathology*, McGraw-Hill, 1951.

48. op. cit., Note 1, p. 152.

49. Sayers, S. P., *The Human Context 7*, 1975, pp. 356–9. A review of Szasz, T., *Ideology and Insanity*.

50. Ingleby, J. D., 'Ideology and the human sciences', *The Human Context 2*, 1970, pp. 159–80. Reprinted in Pateman, T., (ed.), *Counter Course*, Penguin, 1972. 'The psychology of child psychology', *The Human Context 5*, 1973, pp. 557–68. Reprinted in Richards, M. P. M., (ed.), *The Integration of the Child into a Social World*, Cambridge University Press, 1974. 'The job psychologists do', in Armistead, N., (ed.), *Reconstructing Social Psychology*, Penguin, 1974.

51. See Note 44.

52. Illich, I., *Medical Nemesis*, Calder and Boyars, 1975.

53. Waitzkin, H., and Waterman, B., *The Exploitation of Illness in a Capitalist Society*, Bobbs-Merrill, 1974.

54. op. cit., Note 45.

II. Interpretative approaches to psychiatry

1. cf. Taylor, C., 'Interpretation and the sciences of man', *Review of Metaphysics 25*, 1971, pp. 4–51.

2. cf. Giddens, A., *New Rules of Sociological Method*, Hutchinson, 1976.

3. cf. Brown, G. W., 'The family of the schizophrenic patient', in Coppen, A., and Walk, A., *Recent Developments in Schizophrenia*, Royal Medico-Psychological Association, 1967.

4. Laing, R. D., and Esterson, A., *Sanity, Madness and the Family: Families of Schizophrenics*, Tavistock, 1964; Penguin, 1970.

5. See Orford, J., *The Social Psychology of Mental Disorder*, Penguin, 1976, for a survey of this work.

6. Clare, A., *Psychiatry in Dissent: Controversial Issues in Thought and Practice*, Tavistock, 1976.

7. Laing, R. D., *The Divided Self*, Tavistock, 1960; Penguin, 1965. *The Self and Others, Tavistock*, 1961; Penguin, 1971.

8. Pateman, T., 'Sanity, madness and the problem of knowledge', *Radical Philosophy 1*, 1972.

9. Habermas, J., 'On systematically distorted communication', *Inquiry 13*, 1970, pp. 205–18. Reprinted in Drietzel, H.-P., (ed), *Recent Sociology 2*, Collier-Macmillan, 1970.

10. Wing, J. K., *New Society 84*, 7 May 1974, pp. 23–4. A review of Laing, R. D., and Esterson, A., *Sanity, Madness and the Family*.

11. Esterson, A., *The Leaves of Spring*, Tavistock, 1970; Penguin, 1972.

12. Mannoni, M., *The Child, his Illness, and the Family*, Tavistock, 1969; Penguin, 1973.

13. Stierlin, H., *Separating Parents and Adolescents*, Quadrangle, 1974.

14. Deleuze, G., and Guattari, F., *L'Anti-Oedipe*, Editions de Minuit, 1972; English trans., Viking, 1977.

15. Jacoby, R., *Social Amnesia: A Critique of Contemporary Psychology*, Beacon Press, 1975.

16. Busfield, J., 'Family ideology and family pathology', in Armistead, N., (ed.), *Reconstructing Social Psychology*, Penguin, 1974.

17. Fanon, F., *The Wretched of the Earth*, Penguin, 1967; *Black Skins, White Masks*, Paladin, 1970.

18. Sennett, R., and Cobb, J., *The Hidden Injuries of Class*, Vintage, 1973.

19. Brown, G. W., and Harris, T., *Social Origins of Depression*, Tavistock, 1978.

20. Kastenbaum, R., 'Theoretical models and model theoreticians in gerontology', in Kent, D. P., Kastenbaum, R., and Sherwood, S., (eds.), *Research, Planning and Action for the Elderly*, Behavioural Publications, 1970.

21. Ingleby, J. D., 'The psychology of child psychology', *The Human Context 5*, 1973, pp. 557–68. Reprinted in Richards, M. P. M., (ed.), *The Integration of the Child into a Social World*, Cambridge University Press, 1974.

22. Maucorps, P., 'Social vacuum', *The Human Context 2*, 1970, pp. 31–9.

23. Henry, J., *Culture against Man*, Tavistock, 1966.

24. Goffman, E., *Asylums*, Anchor, 1961; Penguin, 1968.

25. Rosenhahn, D. L., 'On being sane in insane places', *Science 179*, 1973, pp. 250–58.

26. Wing, J., and Brown, G., *Institutionalism and Schizophrenia*, Cambridge University Press, 1970.
27. Scheff, T., *Being Mentally Ill: A Sociological Theory*, Weidenfeld and Nicolson, 1966.
28. Balint, M., *The Doctor, his Patient and the Illness*, International University Press, 1957.
29. Pasamanick, B., 'A survey of mental disease in an urban population: IV. An approach to total prevalence rates', *Archives of General Psychiatry 5*, 1961, pp. 151–5.
30. Lemert, E. M., *Social Pathology*, McGraw-Hill, 1951.
31. Becker, H. S., *Outsiders*, Free Press of Glencoe, 1963.
32. Rosenthal, R., and Jacobson, L., *Pygmalion in the Classroom*, Holt, 1968.
33. Hesse, M., 'Theory and value in the social sciences', in Hookway, C., and Pettit, P., (eds.), *Action and Interpretation*, Cambridge University Press, 1978.
34. Goffman, E., 'Mental symptoms and public order', in *Interaction Ritual*, Penguin, 1972.
35. Cooper, D., *The Language of Madness: Explorations in the Hinterland of Revolution*.
36. Sedgwick, P., 'Mental illness *is* illness', *Salmagundi 20*, 1973, pp. 196–224; 'R. D. Laing: Self, symptom and society', in Boyers, R., and Orrill, R., (eds.), *Laing and Anti-Psychiatry*, Penguin, 1974.
37. Mitchell, J., *Psychoanalysis and Feminism*, Penguin, 1975.
38. Gleiss, I., 'Der konservative Gehalt der Anti-Psychiatrie', *Das Argument 17*, 1975, pp. 31–51.
39. op. cit., Note 15.
40. Cited in Laing, R. D., *The Politics of the Family*, Penguin, 1975.
41. McGuire, W., (ed.), *The Freud/Jung Letters*, Hogarth and Routledge & Kegan Paul, 1973.
42. op. cit., Note 31.
43. Sayers, S., 'The concept of mental illness', *Radical Philosophy 5*, 1973, pp. 2–8.
44. Marcuse, H., *Eros and Civilization*, Beacon Press, 1966.
45. Eysenck, H. J., *Uses and Abuses of Psychology*, Penguin, 1953.
46. Rycroft, C., 'Causes and meaning', in *Psychoanalysis Observed*, Constable, 1966.
47. Lacan, J., *Ecrits*, Editions de Seuil, 1966; English trans., Tavistock, 1977.
48. Merleau-Ponty, M., *Phénoménologie de la perception*, Gaillimard, 1945; English trans., *Phenomenology of Perception*, Routledge & Kegan Paul, 1961.
49. Lorenzer, A., *Sprachzerstörung und Rekonstruktion*, Suhrkamp, 1971.

50. Ricoeur, P., *Freud and Philosophy*, Yale University Press, 1970.
51. Szasz, T., *The Myth of Mental Illness*, Harper and Row, 1961; Paladin, 1972.
52. Shafer, R., *A New Language for Psychoanalysis*, Yale University Press, 1976.
53. Laing, R. D., *The Self and Others*, Tavistock, 1961; Penguin, 1971.
54. op. cit., Note 47.
55. Coulter, J., *Approaches to Insanity*, Martin Robertson, 1973.
56. op. cit., Note 50.
57. Popper, K., *Conjectures and Refutations*, Routledge & Kegan Paul, 1963.
58. op. cit., Note 45.
59. Borger, R., and Cioffi, F., *Explanation in the Behavioural Sciences*, Cambridge University Press, 1970.
60. Cosin, B. R., Freeman, C. F., and Freeman, N. H., 'Critical empiricism criticised: The case of Freud', *J. Theory Soc. Behaviour 1*, 1971, pp. 121–49.
61. op. cit., Note 52.
62. Althusser, L., *Lenin and Philosophy and Other Essays*, New Left Books, 1971.
63. Lacan, see Note 47.
64. op. cit., Note 50.
65. Habermas, J., *Erkenntnis und Interesse*, Suhrkamp, 1968; English trans., *Knowledge and Human Interests*, Heinemann, 1972.
66. See e.g. Wollheim, R., (ed.), *Freud: A Collection of Critical Essays*, Anchor, 1974.
67. Fisher, S., and Greenberg, R. P., *The Scientific Credibility of Freud's Theories*, Harvester, 1977.
68. Ingleby, J. D., 'The politics of depth psychology', in Broughton, J. M., (ed.), *Critical Developmental Psychology* (forthcoming).
69. Deleuze and Guattari; see Note 14.
70. op. cit., Note 15.
71. See Hesse, M., *The Structure of Scientific Inference*, Macmillan, 1974.

2. The American Mental Health Industry

1. James, William, *The Varieties of Religious Experience*, Lectures IV–V, passim, New American Library, Mentor paperback, 1958.
2. Hale, Nathan G., Jr, *Freud and the Americans, Vol. I (1876–1917)*, New York, Oxford, 1971. This work provides a detailed summary of considerable scholarly importance, albeit without critical historical analysis; cf. also Deutsch, Albert, *The Mentally Ill in America*, New York, Columbia, 1949.
3. cf. Marx, Karl, *Grundrisse*, trans., M. Nicolaus, Penguin, 1973, pp.

701–12. For a general survey based upon a slightly different definition, cf. Baran, Paul, and Sweezy, Paul, *Monopoly Capital*, New York, Monthly Review Press; Penguin, 1968.

4. This is consistent with our definition, insofar as the legitimation of the social order may require many reform measures on behalf of people. Obviously a certain amount of welfare must be provided so people can continue to buy commodities, provide a reserve supply of labor and not grow so disaffected that they may entertain revolutionary ideas. In addition, the state will come to represent some portion of the reaction to capital, as well as certain semi-autonomous functions, such as the courts. All this is of no present concern. However, as the state will enter again and again in our discussion, it is well to bear in mind some of its complexities.

5. For a discussion that focuses upon advertising, cf. Ewen, Stuart, *Captains of Consciousness*, New York, McGraw-Hill, 1976.

6. Baran and Sweezy, op. cit., Note 3, Penguin, pp. 215–43.

7. For some aspects of the history of this boundary, see Foucault, Michel, *Madness and Civilization*, New York, Pantheon, 1965; also Rosen, George, *Madness in Society*, New York, Harper Torchbook, 1969.

8. Albert Deutsch, op. cit., Note 2, pp. 300–331.

9. It is of considerable interest to observe that the state of psychiatric incarceration in the late nineteenth century was itself something of a regression from a previous reformist phase in which *early* capitalist relations had been employed to bring things up to date. As David Rothman pointed out in his *The Discovery of the Asylum*, (Boston, Little Brown, 1971), the Jacksonian era of reform had extended to asylums in a striking way. A frenzy of order descended upon the mental patient: severe, geometrically designed buildings, extraordinary attention paid to carving up the day into detailed segments of time, an intense puritanical moralization – all the cultural innovations entailed in the imposition of a temporally ordered work discipline (cf. Thompson, E. P., 'Time, Work-Discipline and Industrial Capitalism', *Past and Present 38*, 1967, pp. 56–93), were turned to the 'cure' of madness. A certain benefit resulted, to be sure, from the very attention directed toward the inmates; but when the cure was not forthcoming, society lost interest and let the asylums sink into the slough from which Beers and his movement sought to rescue them half a century later. At a deeper level, it may be speculated that the impetus for this type of reform died down (although it must be emphasized that, as with all early cultural formations, its lineaments can be found in all that followed) because of a dawning awareness of the obsolescence of quantitative labor-power, coupled with the rise of other, more consuming crises of reform, such as the mid-century struggle over slavery.

10. The movement had opened its arms from the beginning. Its initial

statement of goals listed as the first priority (i.e., *before* that of raising the standard of care for those already insane): 'To work for the protection of the mental health of the public', and vowed 'to enlist the aid of the Federal Government so far as may seem desirable; to coordinate existing agencies . . .' etc. (Deutsch, op. cit., Note 2.)

11. It is of interest to note that the ubiquitous Dr Salmon introduced yet another dimension to the meaning of mental health in America by psychologically examining immigrants at Ellis Island as early as 1904 (cf. Chu, Franklin, D., and Trotter, Sharland, *The Madness Establishment*, New York, Grossman, 1974). Undoubtedly, the influx of immigrants with their strange, unassimilable ways heightened American sensitivity to the need for defining 'healthy' standards of behavior.

12. Deutsch, op. cit., Note 2, pp. 309–10.

13. For further reflections on dirt as it pertains to money, capitalism and racism, see my *White Racism: a Psychohistory*, New York, Pantheon, 1970.

14. Aronowitz, Stanley, *False Promises*, New York, McGraw-Hill, 1973.

15. Not surprisingly, this function came into its heyday in the 1920s. It is also noteworthy that the comparison was drawn with wartime psychiatry, the worker and the soldier being correctly identified as victims of combat fatigue and shellshock, without considering the actual antagonism in which the former was engaged. As might be expected, industrial psychiatry waned during the Depression of the 1930s. Since the Second War it has been relatively subsumed into the general proliferation of mental health services and psychotherapeutics.

16. Consider the following, from the *New York Times* of 8 November 1976. Headlined 'Doctor Terms Handguns A Public Health Problem', the article cites a report in *The Journal of the American Medical Association*, in which an Oregon psychiatrist, Dr Charles H. Browning, claims that 'The prevention of avoidable or unnecessary deaths, injuries, or illness should be a major goal of physicians.' The article notes that 'despite deaths and injuries from handguns . . . there have been no attempts to control them as a public health measure'. Today handguns, tomorrow nuclear war. Meantime a battle has been hotly waged in California concerning the setting up, under the auspices of psychiatrist Louis Jolyn West, of a $1.5 million Center for the Reduction of Violence, one of the main functions of which would be to develop mass-screening tests for the detection (and possible psychosurgery) of (sic) violence-prone individuals. Though currently shelved as a result of heavy protest, no sensible person considers that the last of such proposals has been seen.

17. This is not the place to give the topic the attention it deserves; but to avoid misunderstanding, it should be emphasized that I am not denying

the objective reality of distinctions in emotional disturbances, nor that some portion of them, including, for example, schizophrenia, is structurally affected by organic dispositions the investigation of which requires conceptions drawn from natural science. The point is only that the task is in fact blocked by the prevalent use of a model crudely drawn from somatic disease. That official psychiatry expends so much effort on diagnosis is only the sign of the model's inadequacy.

18. There is no quicker way for an outside observer to be convinced of this statement than to peruse any of the official psychiatric journals. The experience is by and large chilling. A dialectic is at work in these publications according to which the strength of a contribution varies directly with its approximation to sterile scientistic jargon and inversely with its social relevance. Thus certain types of problems, especially quantifiable drug studies, get gala treatment (all the more so as drug ads are a main source of revenue), while anything of real human interest is either banalized or suppressed. As an indication of how the profession tries to preoccupy itself, one may turn to a quasi-scientific newsletter with a blue-ribbon advisory board of psychiatrists, distributed free of charge to all psychiatrists and financed by – guess what! – drug ads. A rough content analysis of one of these publications, *Clinical Psychiatry News*, for October 1976, discloses the following distribution of topics: 6 articles on the politics of practice (malpractice, the ways of hospitals, etc.); 5 on various biological discoveries; 5 on biological forms of treatment such as drugs; 5 on hypnosis (which is evidently making a comeback); 5 on behavioral analyses, including diagnosis; 3 on psychotherapy (two of which debunk it, the third being gibberish); 2 on parapsychology; and 1 on a 'socially relevant' topic. The content of the latter is as revealing as its number, the point being that feminists have better sex but more unstable marriages than ordinary women, and the conclusion, that negotiation rather than dominance should be the rule in marriage.

19. Freud, S., *The Future of Illusion, Standard Edition*, Vol XXI, p. 12.

20. op. cit., Note 2.

21. It should be recalled that Freud's most 'progressive' essay, 'Civilized Sexual Morality and Modern Nervous Illness' (SE, 9, 179), was written in 1908.

22. op. cit., Note 2, p. 345.

23. op. cit., Note 5.

24. It should be kept in mind here that psychoanalysis in particular, and psychiatry in general, has, for obvious reasons, mainly been an urban pursuit, and located in the biggest cities at that. Indeed, New York City alone contains approximately half the psychoanalytic population of the United States. In recent years there has tended to be a diffusion

outward to big-city suburban areas and smaller cities. Rural regions in general cannot support a psychiatric/psychoanalytic population; nor does emotional difficulty tend to get put into psychological categories there.

25. cf. *The Question of Lay Analysis*, SE, *20*, 179, which was written – futilely – to persuade American colleagues.

26. Fenichel, Otto, 'The Drive to Amass Wealth', *Psychoanalytic Quarterly*, Vol. VII, 1938, pp. 69–95.

27. Chu and Trotter, op. cit., Note 11.

28. In some state institutions, for example, psychiatric nurses have gained power. One even became director for a while of Bronx Psychiatric Center, one of the institutions (a state hospital) most affected by the community movement.

29. Chu and Trotter, op. cit., Note 11; Duhl, Leonard J., and Leopold, Robert L., *Mental Health and Urban Social Policy*, San Francisco, Jossey-Bass, 1969.

30. Kaplan, Seymour R., and Roman, Melvin, *The Organization and Delivery of Mental Health Services in the Ghetto: The Lincoln Experience*, New York, Praeger, 1973.

31. For example, Grunebaum, H., ed., *The Practice of Community Mental Health*, Boston, Little-Brown, 1970; a large and supposedly comprehensive collection, has much to do with 'the poor', but contains no meaningful mention of social class. At one point (p. 749) a community is defined as 'a group of persons who live within a defined area'.

32. In another variation of the social obtuseness characteristic of American psychiatry, a number of the earlier excursions into community mental health were designed as replicas of Maxwell Jones' pathbreaking English ventures, leaving out of account that an American urban ghetto did not have quite the same structure or cohesiveness as an English country village. To these minds, one catchment area was as good as another, both being essentially a matter of a certain number of people.

33. For systems theory, see Bateson, Gregory, *Steps to an Ecology of Mind*, New York, Ballantine Books, 1972; Gray William, Duhl, Frederick J., and Rizzo, Nicholas D., *General Systems Theory and Psychiatry*, Boston, Little-Brown, 1969; for family and group therapy, see Boszormanzi-Nagy, Ivan, and Framo, James (eds.), *Intensive Family Therapy*, New York, Harper and Row, 1965; Sager, Clifford J., and Kaplan, Helen Singer (eds.), *Progress in Group and Family Therapy*, New York, Brunner-Mazel, 1972; cf. also Kovel, Joel, *A Complete Guide to Therapy*, New York, Pantheon, 1976.

34. Speck, Ross and Attneave, Carolyn, *Family Networks*, New York, Pantheon, 1973.

35. The magazine *Psychology Today*, for example, regularly takes out full-page newspaper ads to draw advertising. In these ads, it crows

that it is the genuine wave of the times, and that its 4,000,000 sub-scribers represent today's ideal-type of the narcissistically perfect individual who buys the goods early and often.

36. Kovel, op. cit., Note 33; Jacoby, Russell, *Social Amnesia*, Boston, Beacon, 1975.

37. In this respect it should be noted that older therapies, including psycho-analysis, are not exempt from the trends mentioned here. Indeed the breakup into endless factions and schools is often carried on in pre-cisely this spirit. If there is resistance within psychoanalysis to the trend, it lies in the therapeutic caution which attends taking the un-conscious seriously.

38. For example, *est*, one of the most successful of the recent wave of ther-apies, has, along with its progressive intentions, a highly bureaucratic organizational structure that requires scrutiny: cf. Kornbluth, Jesse, 'The Führer Over est', *New Times*, Vol. 6, No. 6, 19 March 1976, pp. 36–52.

39. For an account of how TA is used by the Internal Revenue Service for their training programme, see Klee, Earl, 'Serving Time with the I.R.S.', *Social Policy*, Vol. 5, March–April 1975, pp. 43–8.

40. cf. Jacoby, op. cit., Note 36, Chapter VII.

41. Szasz, Thomas, *Law, Liberty and Psychiatry*, New York, Macmillan, 1963.

42. Brown, Phil, *Toward a Marxist Psychology*, New York, Harper & Row, 1974; Agel, Jerome, (ed.), *The Radical Therapist*, New York, Ballantine, 1971.

43. Chavkin, Samuel, 'Therapy or Mind Control? Congress Endorses Psychosurgery', *The Nation*, 23 October 1976, pp. 398–402.

44. The immediate issue concerned solidarity with other house officers and staff physicians over recognition of a bargaining agent in contract negotiations with medical schools and the financially wracked City of New York. Although this struggle did not go beyond first stages, it forced these doctors to consider the novel possibility of an identity of interest between themselves, other hospital workers, and patients.

3. On the Medicalization of Deviance and Social Control

1. Illich, Ivan, *Medical Nemesis*, New York, Pantheon, 1976. See also Zola, Irving K., 'Medicine as an Institution of Social Control', *Socio-logical Review 20*, 1972, pp. 487–504, and Fox, Renée C., 'The Medi-calization and Demedicalization of American Society', *Daedalus 106*: 1, Winter 1977, pp. 9–22.

2. For a more complete conceptual and historical analysis of the medi-calization of deviance see Conrad, Peter, and Schneider, Joseph W., *Deviance: From Badness to Sickness*, St Louis, C. V. Mosby, 1980.

3. *Webster's New Ideal Dictionary*, Springfield, Mass., G. and C. Merriam Company, 1973.

4. For example, see special issues *The Hastings Center Studies* 1:3, 1973, and *The Journal of Medicine and Philosophy* 1:3, September 1973.

5. Kass, Leon R., 'Regarding the End of Medicine and the Pursuit of Health', *The Public Interest 40*, Summer 1975, pp. 11–42.

6. Cited in Febrega, Horacio, and Manning, Peter K., 'Disease, Illness, and Deviant Careers', in Scott, Robert A., and Douglas, Jack D., (eds.), *Theoretical Perspectives on Deviance*, New York, Basic Books, 1972, pp. 93–116.

7. Cited in Mechanic, David, *Medical Sociology*, New York, Free Press, 1968, p. 16.

8. Dubos, Rene, *Mirage of Health*, New York, Harper, 1959.

9. Sedgwick, Peter, 'Illness – Mental and Otherwise', *Hastings Center Studies* 1:3, 1973, p. 30.

10. ibid.

11. Sedgwick, op. cit., Note 9, p. 31.

12. Freidson, Eliot, *The Profession of Medicine*, New York, Dodd Mead, 1970, pp. 214–15.

13. I cannot think of any illness designations that are positive judgments or any illness conditions that are viewed as desirable states.

14. Freidson, op. cit., Note 12, p. 223.

15. Parsons, Talcott, *The Social System*, Glencoe, Ill., Free Press, 1951, pp. 428–79.

16. There have been a number of critiques and modifications of the sick role. See for example Gerald Gordon, *Role Theory and Illness*, New Haven, Conn., College and University Press, 1966; Mechanic, op. cit., Note 7; Miriam Sieger and Humphrey Osmond, *Models of Madness, Models of Medicine*, New York, Macmillan, 1947; and Talcott Parsons, 'The Sick Role and the Role of the Physician Reconsidered', *Health and Society*, Summer 1975, pp. 257–77.

17. Durkheim, Emile, *The Division of Labor in Society*, New York, Free Press, 1933 (1893).

18. Kitterie, Nicholas, *The Right to Be Different*, Baltimore, Johns Hopkins Press, 1971.

19. Rieff, Philip, *The Triumph of the Therapeutic*, New York, Harper and Row, 1966.

20. Quoted in Blumgart, Herman L., 'Caring For the Patient', *New England Journal of Medicine 270*, 1964, p. 449.

21. For an instructive analysis of the predominance of *social* changes in the 'conquest' of communicable diseases, see Dubos, op. cit., Note 8.

22. Freidson, op. cit., p. 251.

23. Reiff, op. cit., Note 12.

24. For mental illness, see Foucault, Michel, *Madness and Civilization*,

New York, Pantheon, 1965; and Szasz, Thomas, *Manufacture of Madness*, New York, Dell, 1970; for public health, see Rosen, George, 'The Evolution of Social Medicine', in Freeman, H. E., Levine, S., and Reeder, L. (eds.), *Handbook of Medical Sociology*, Englewood Cliffs, New Jersey, Prentice-Hall, 1972.

25. For alcoholism, see Trice, Harrison M., and Roman, Paul M., *Spirits and Demons at Work*, Ithaca, New York, New York State School of Industrial Relations, 1972; Gusfield, Joseph R., 'Moral Passage: The Symbolic Process in Public Designations of Deviance', *Social Problems 15*, 1967, pp. 175–88; for drug addiction, see Nelkin, Dorothy, *Methadone Maintenance: A Technological Fix*, New York, Braziller, 1973; for hyperactive children, see Conrad, Peter, 'The Discovery of Hyperkinesis; Notes on the Medicalization of Deviant Behavior', *Social Problems 23:1*, 1975, pp. 12–21; Conrad Peter, *Identifying Hyperactive Children: The Medicalization of Deviant Behavior*, Lexington, Mass., D. C. Heath, 1976; for suicide, see Atkinson, J. Maxwell, 'Societal Reactions to Suicide: The Role of Coroners' Definitions', in Cohen, Stanley, *Images of Deviance*, Baltimore, Penguin, 1971; for obesity, see Szasz, Thomas, *Ceremonial Chemistry*, New York, Doubleday, 1974; for crime, see Moran, Richard, 'Biomedical research and the politics of crime control: a historical perspective', *Contemporary Crises 2*, 1977, pp. 335–57; for violence, see Coleman, Lee S., 'Perspectives on Medical Research on Violence', *American Journal of Orthopsychiatry 44*, October 1974, pp. 675–87; for child abuse, see Gelles, Richard J., 'The Social Construction of Child Abuse', *American Journal of Orthopsychiatry 45*, April 1975, pp. 363–73; for learning problems, see Schrag, Peter, and Divoky, Diane, *The Myth of the Hyperactive Child*, New York, Pantheon, 1975.

26. This has been viewed as humanitarian and scientific progress by many; indeed, it often leads to 'humanitarian and scientific' treatment rather than punishment as a response to deviant behavior. However, there have also been criticisms of medicalization; cf. Kitterie, op. cit., Note 18; Szasz, op. cit., Notes 24 and 25; Conrad, op. cit., Note 25; and Zola, Irving K., 'In the Name of Health: On Some Socio-Political Consequences of Medical Influence', *Social Science and Medicine 9*, 1975, pp. 83–7.

27. op. cit., Note 25, p. 149.

28. Kitterie, op. cit., Note 18.

29. Pitts, Jesse, 'Social Control: The Concept', in Sills, David (ed.), *International Encyclopedia of Social Sciences*, no. 14, New York, Macmillan, 1968; see also Mechanic, David, 'Health and Illness In Technological Societies', in *The Hasting Center Studies 1:3*, 1973, pp. 7–18.

30. Laufer, Maurice W., Denhoff, Eric, and Solomons, Gerald, 'The

Hyperkinetic Impulse Disorder in Children's Behavior Problems', *Psychosomatic Medicine 19*, 1957, pp. 38–49; for reviews from a general medical perspective see Wender, Paul, *Minimal Brain Dysfunction in Children*, New York, Wiley, 1971; and Safer, Daniel J., and Allen, Richard P., *Hyperactive Children: Diagnosis and Management*, Baltimore, University Park Press, 1976; two excellent critical articles are Scroufe, Alan J., and Stewart, Mark, 'Treating Problem Children with Stimulant Drugs', *New England Journal of Medicine 289*, 1973, pp. 407–21; and Rie, Herbert E., 'Hyperactivity in Children', *American Journal of Diseases in Children 129*, July 1975, pp. 783–9.

31. See for example Becker, Howard S., *The Outsiders*, New York, Free Press, 1963; Erikson, Kai T., 'Notes on the Sociology of Deviance', *Social Problems 9*, 1962, p. 307–14; Kitsuse, John, 'Societal Reactions to Deviant Behavior: Problems in Theory and Method', *Social Problems 9*, 1962, pp. 247–56; and Schur, Edwin, *Labeling Deviant Behavior*, New York, Harper and Row, 1971.

32. While doing participant observation research at a pediatric diagnostic hyperactivity clinic, I noticed that very few children from parochial schools were referred for hyperactivity. In fact, two children were referred for hyperactivity after they were transferred to public school; two other parents were considering sending their children to parochial school as 'treatment' for their hyperactivity. Eleanor Maccoby reports finding no hyperactive children in schoolrooms in the People's Republic of China; cf. 'Impressions from China', *Society for Research in Child Development Newsletter*, Autumn, 1974, p. 5.

33. Bradley, Charles A., 'The Behavior of Children Receiving Benzedrine', *American Journal of Psychiatry 94*, March, 1937, pp. 577–85.

34. Fox, Richard G., 'The XYZ offender: A Modern Myth?' *Journal of Criminal Law, Criminology and Police Science 62*, 1971, pp. 1–15.

35. Dennis Dubey, after a critical evaluation of research, concludes:

The evidence taken as a whole does not strongly support the notion that organic factors play a significant role in the behavior problems of most hyperactive children. The results from biochemical studies and studies of severe pregnancy and birth complications are clearly negative; results from electroencephalographic and neurological studies are conflicting; genetic studies are plagued by methodological difficulties. As such, the assumption that a hyperkinetic child suffers from minimal brain dysfunction or any other biological deviation is unwarranted in the absence of unequivocal data. For most hyperkinetic children, such data is unavailable.

Dubey, Dennis, 'Organic Factors in Hyperkinesis: A Critical Evaluation', *American Journal of Orthopsychiatry 46*, April, 1976, pp. 353–66.

36. See 'The Social Construction of Hyperactivity: Uncertainty and Medical Diagnosis', in Conrad, op. cit., Note 25, pp. 51–70.

37. Office of Child Development, 'Report of the Conference on the Use

of Stimulant Drugs in Treatment of Behaviorally Disturbed Children',
Washington, D.C., Department of Health, Education and Welfare,
1971; Joint Committee of the American Bar Association, *Drug Addiction: Crime or Disease?*, Bloomington, Indiana, University of Indiana
Press, 1960; Chavkin, Samuel, 'Therapy or Mind Control? Congress
Endorses Psychosurgery', *The Nation*, October, 1976, pp. 398–402.
38. Radelate, Michael M., 'Medical Hegemony as Social Control: The use
of Tranquilizers', paper presented at meetings of Society for the Study
of Social Problems, September 1977; on drug industry, see Goddard,
James L., 'The Medical Business', *Scientific American*, September 1973;
and Silverman, Milton, and Lee, Philip, *Pills, Profits and Politics*,
Berkeley, University of California Press, 1974; on the drug industry
and hyperactivity, see Charles, Alan, 'The Case of Ritalin', *New Republic*, 23 October 1971, pp. 17–19; and Hentoff, Nat, 'Drug Pushing in
the Schools: The Professionals', *The Village Voice*, May 1972, pp.
21–3.
39. Trice and Roman, op. cit., Note 25, p. 11.
40. Conrad and Schneider, op. cit., Note 2, Chapter 8.
41. See for example, Medvedev, Roy, and Medvedev, Zhores, *A Question
of Madness*, New York, Random House, 1972; and *Abuse of Psychiatry for Political Repression*, Vol. II, Washington, D.C., United States
Government Printing Office, 1975.
42. Zola, op. cit., Note 26, p. 182.

4. Towards a Critical History of the Psychiatric Profession

1. Watzlawick, P., et al., *Change*, Norton, 1974.
2. Eysenck, H. J., 'The effects of psychotherapy: an evaluation', *Journal
of Consulting Psychology 16*, 1952, pp. 319–24.
3. Eysenck, H. J., *The Future of Psychiatry*, Methuen, 1975.
4. Goldie, N., 'The division of labour among the mental health professions – a negotiated or an imposed order'. Paper presented to B.S.A.
Conference, Manchester, April 1976.
5. Goldie, N., 'Eclecticism as the dominant ideology and its contribution
towards the maintenance of the status quo in British psychiatry', in
press.
6. Clare, A., *Psychiatry in Dissent*, Tavistock, 1976.
7. ibid., p, 69.
8. Cited in Rachman, S. J., and Philips, C., *Psychology and Medicine*,
Temple Smith, 1975.
9. Will, D., 'Four issues in psychotherapy training', in Walton, H., (Chair-
man), *Proceedings of a conference on the Teaching of Psychotherapy*,
published by the Association of University Teachers of Psychiatry,
1976.

10. Clare, A., in *Nursing Mirror*, 1978. A review of *Psychiatry Observed*.
11. Ackernecht, E. H., *Therapeutics*, Hafner, 1973.
12. Smail, D., 'Clinical psychology and the medical model', *Bull. Br. Psychol. Soc. 26*, 1973, pp. 211–14.
13. Scull, A. T., 'Museums of madness: the social organization of insanity in nineteenth century England', unpublished Ph.D. dissertation, Princeton University, 1974; 'From madness to mental illness: : medical men as moral entrepreneurs', *Archives Européennes de Sociologie 16*, 1975, pp. 218–61; 'Mad-doctors and magistrates. English Psychiatry's struggle for professional autonomy in the nineteenth century', *Archives Européennes de Sociologie 17*, 1976, pp. 279–305; *Decarceration*, Prentice Hall, 1977. See also *Museums of Madness*, Allen Lane, 1979.
14. Wing, J. K., *Reasoning about Madness*, Oxford, 1978.
15. Scull, A. T., 'From madness to mental illness . . .' See Note 13.
16. Cited by Scull, op. cit., Note 15.
17. Scull, A. T., 'Mad-doctors and magistrates . . .' See Note 13.
18. Freidson, E., *Profession of Medicine*, Dodd Mead and Co., 1970; *Professional Dominance*, Atherton, 1970.
19. Waitzkin, H. B., and Waterman, B., *The Exploitation of Illness in Capitalist Society*, Bobbs-Merrill, 1974.
20. Skultans, V., *Madness and Morals*, Routledge & Kegan Paul, 1975.
21. Hofstadter, R., *Social Darwinism in American Thought*, Braziller, 1965.
22. Baruch, G., and Treacher, A., *Psychiatry Observed*, Routledge & Kegan Paul, 1978.
23. op. cit., Note 17, p. 303.
24. Ewins, D., 'The origins of the compulsory commitment provisions of the Mental Health Act (1959)'. Unpublished M.A. thesis, University of Sheffield, 1974.
25. Rosen, G., 'The evolution of social medicine', in Freeman, H. E., et al., *Handbook of Medical Sociology*, Prentice Hall, 2nd edn 1972, p. 34.
26. ibid., p. 45.
27. Illich, I., *Medical Nemesis*, Calder and Boyars, 1975.
28. Riese, W., 'The structure of the clinical history', *Bull. Hist. Med. 16*, 1944, pp. 437–49.
29. op. cit., Note 14.
30. Parsons, T., *The Social System*, Free Press, 1951.
31. op. cit., Note 19.
32. Semmel, B., *Imperialism and Social Reform*, Allen and Unwin, 1960.
33. ibid.
34. op. cit., Note 24, p. 41.
35. ibid., p. 51.
36. op. cit., Note 22.
37. Scull, A. T., *Decarceration*. See Note 13.

38. Wing, J. K., and Brown, G. W., *Institutionalism and Schizophrenia*, Cambridge University Press, 1970.
39. Gostin, L. O., *A Human Condition*, vols I and II, *Mind*, London, 1977.
40. Michaels, R. M., and Sevitt, M. A., 'The patient and the first psychiatric interview', *Brit. J. Psychiat. 132*, 1978, pp. 288–92.
41. Illich, I., et al., *Disabling Professions*, Marion Boyars, 1977.
42. Sedgwick, P., 'Mental illness *is* illness', *Salmagundi 20*, 1973, pp. 196–224.
43. Morgan, D., 'Explaining mental illness', *Archives Européennes de Sociologie 16*, 1975, pp. 262–80.
44. Scott, R. D., 'The treatment barrier', *Brit. J. Med. Psychol 46*, 1973, pp. 45–67; Scott, R. D., and Ashworth, P. L., 'The "axis value" and the transfer of psychosis', *Brit. J. Med. Psychol. 38*, 1965, pp. 97–116; Scott, R. D., and Ashworth, P. L., ' "Closure" at the first schizophrenic breakdown: a family study', *Brit. J. Med. Psychol. 40*, 1967, pp. 109–45; Scott, R. D., and Ashworth, P. L., 'The shadow of the ancestor: a historical factor in the transmission of schizophrenia', *Brit. J. Med. Psychol. 42*, 1969, pp. 13–32; Scott, R. D., Ashworth, P. L., and Casson, P. D., 'Violation of parental role structure and outcome in schizophrenia', *Soc. Sci. Med 4*, 1970, pp. 41–64.
45. Mechanic, D., *Mental Health and Social Policy*, Prentice Hall, 1969.
46. Scott, R. D., 'The treatment barrier'. See Note 44.
47. op. cit., Note 22.
48. Cited by Jones, K., *The History of the Mental Health Services*, Routledge & Kegan Paul, 1972.

5. French Anti-psychiatry

1. In France there was no independent discipline of psychiatry until after 1968: the emergence of an independent psychiatric specialty was one of the results of the May–June 1968 revolt. Before 1968 all French psychiatrists were neuropsychiatrists.
2. Recamier, P. C., Lebovici, Serge, Paumelle, Philippe, and Diatkine, Rene, *Le Psychanalyste sans divan*, Paris, Payot, 1970.
3. Lacan, Jacques, *Ecrits*, Paris, Seuil, 1966, p. 176.
4. Deleuze, Gilles, and Guattari, Félix, *L'Anti-Oedipe: Capitalisme et Schizophrénie*, Paris, Editions de Minuit, 1972. English Edition: *Anti-Oedipus: Capitalism and Schizophrenia*, New York, Viking, 1977. All citations will be from the English translation.
5. The context for this quote is Lacan's description of how the child 'makes' himself in his own image in the mirror:

'This jubilant assumption of his mirror-image by the little man, at the *infans* stage, still sunk in his motor incapacity and nurseling dependency, would seem to exhibit in an exemplary situation the symbolic matrix in which the *I* is precipitated in a primordial form, before it is objectified in the dialectic of identification with the other, and before language restores to it, in the universal, its function as subject ... But the important point is that this form situates the instance of the *ego*, before its social determination, in a fictional direction, which will always remain irreducible for the individual alone, or rather, which will only rejoin the development of the subject asymptotically, whatever the success of the dialectical synthesis by which he must resolve as *I* his disaccordance with his own reality.'

See Lacan, Jacques, 'The mirror-phase as Formative of the Function of the I'. Trans. Roussel, Jean, *New Left Review*, No. 51, September–October 1968, pp. 73–83. This essay is a translation of a paper read to the international Congress of Psychoanalysis at Marienbad in 1949 and is published in Lacan's *Ecrits*. A good discussion in English of the implications of Lacan's mirror phase for the development of the psyche is to be found in Mitchell, Juliet, *Psychoanalysis and Feminism*, New York, Random House, 1974.

6. Mannoni, Maud, *Le Psychiatre, son 'fou' et la psychanalyse*, Paris, Seuil, 1970, p. 28.

7. Mannoni believes that psychoanalysis is definitionally subversive in terms of how it fragments the 'centered' subject of ego psychology, insisting that the true subject has his words stolen by an ego who is there in order not to hear him.

8. The fact that when Lacan 'uses' linguistics he transforms terms and meanings is a source of contention because it tends to close down psychoanalysis' communication with and criticism from other disciplines. A linguist cannot criticize Lacan on the basis of his understanding of his own field, he must first 'learn' Lacanian.

9. Wittgenstein, *The Tractatus*, New York, Humanities Press, 1963. This idea of using philosophy not to convey explicit 'knowledge', but as a therapeutic vehicle has been developed by the British school of philosophers influenced by Wittgenstein and explicitly formulated as such by Brian Farrel in his paper, 'An Appraisal of Therapeutic Positivism', *Mind*, Vol. LV, Nos. 217, 218, January and April, 1946.

10. Deleuze, Gilles, and Guattari, Félix, *Anti-Oedipus*, p. 1.

11. Typically, Lacan expressed this dual process in a play on words which was the title of his seminar for 1973–4: 'Le Nom du Père'. Le NOM is the father's name which the child accepts as his own along with the father's NON. This dual acceptance permits entrance into the Symbolic dimension.

12. Deleuze and Guattari, *Anti-Oedipus*, p. 55.

13. ibid., p. 54.

14. ibid.
15. It has been often remarked that Deleuze and Guattari's use of the term 'capitalism' may be misleading. They seem really to be referring to complex industrial societies.
16. They take as an example a cure among the African Ndembu which is recounted in the work of anthropologist Victor Turner. See Deleuze and Guattari, *L'Anti-Oedipe*, p. 167.
17. ibid., p. 360.
18. ibid.
19. See Guattari, Félix, 'Micro-politique du désir', in *Psychanalyse et politique*, ed. Armando Verdiglione, Paris, Seuil, 1947, p. 47.
20. In fact some Lacanian *militants* feel that the articulation of psychoanalysis' role in the class struggle will emerge through making the analytic relationship a directly political one, a catalyst for political activism.

    See Bromh, J. M., 'Psychoanalysis and Revolution', *Partisans*, No. 46, February–March 1969; and Boons, M. C., 'Automatisme, compulsion: marques, remarques', *Tel Quel*, No. 42, Summer 1970.
21. See Politzer, Georges, 'Médecine ou philosophie', in Politzer, G., *Ecrits*, *2*, Les Fondements de la Psychologie, Paris, Editions Sociales, 1969, pp. 7–19.
22. See Althusser, Louis, 'Freud et Lacan', *La Nouvelle Critique*, Nos. 161–2, December–January 1964–5, pp. 88–108.
23. Lacan, Jacques, *Ecrits*, p. 833.
24. Misunderstandings of this quite fundamental point can make Lacan's writing seem like nonsense. For example, Lacan often makes the point that 'Il n'y a pas de rapports sexuels' (there are no sexual relations). He is speaking on a symbolic level.
25. See Mitchell, Juliet, *Psychoanalysis and Feminism*.
26. Castel, Robert, *Le Psychanalysme*, Paris, Maspero, 1972, p. 21.
27. Foucault, Michel, *Madness and Civilization: A History of Insanity in the Age of Reason*, New York, Random House, 1965.
28. Castel, *Le Psychanalysme*, p. 22.
29. ibid., p. 23.
30. ibid. The reference to Lacan's Wednesdays is to Lacan's seminar, usually given on Wednesday afternoons to 'le tout Paris'.
31. I conducted interviews with members of several anti-psychiatric groups, as well as with a sample of French psychiatrists and psychoanalysts of all political and analytic persuasions during a field-study of the French psychoanalytic culture which I made in 1973–4. These citations are from that study.
32. 'Au lieu de définir le sujet comme identité autonome, il [Lacan] le définit comme sujet en crise, comme sujet fendu. Le sujet, pour la théorie lacanienne, se définit donc par la fente qui le constitute ...;

l'être du sujet humaniste était solide et évident. L'être du sujet lacanienne est vacillant et en crise.' See *Gardes Fous*, no. 1.

6. Breaking the Circuit of Control

1. Basaglia, Franco (ed.), *L'istituzione negata*, Einaudi, 1968. German trans., *Die negierte Institution oder die Gemeinschaft der Ausgeschlossen*, Suhrkamp, 1971.

7. Report from Norway

1. Szasz, T., *The Myth of Mental Illness*, Harper and Row, 1961.
2. Foucault, M., *Madness and Civilisation*, Tavistock, 1967.
3. op. cit., Note 1.
4. Winnicott, D., *The Maturational Processes and the Facilitating Environment*, Hogarth, 1965.
5. Bion, W., 'A theory of thinking', *Int. J. Psychoanalysis 43*, 1962, pp. 306–10; *Elements of Psycho-analysis*, Heinemann, 1963; *Brazilian Lectures I*, Saõ Paulo, 1973.
6. Meltzer, D., *The Psycho-analytic Process*, Heinemann, 1967; Meltzer, D., et al., *Explorations in Autism*, Clunie Press, 1976; Meltzer, D., *The Kleinian Development*, Clunie Press, 1978.
7. Stierlin, H., *Separating Parents and Adolescents*, Quadrangle, 1974; 'Familie: samspill og generasjonskonflikt', in Haugsgjerd, S., and Engelstad, F., (eds.), *Seks Samtaler om Psykiatri*, Pax Verlag A/S, 1976.
8. Lorenzer, A., *Entworf zu einer materialistischen Sozialisationstheorie*, Suhrkamp, 1972; 'Psykoanalyse og samfunns teori', in Haugsgjerd, S., and Engelstad, F., (eds.), *Seks Samtaler om Psykiatri*, Pax Verlag A/S, 1976.
9. Duve, A. M., *Det første levearets psykologi*, Oslo, 1972.
10. cf. Winnicott, op. cit., Note 4.